Our AI Journey

1st Edition

Our AI Journey

Understanding the AI Revolution and How We Might Shape It to Influence the Future of Human Society

1st Edition

Neil Mayes

Copyright © 2024 Neil Mayes
All rights reserved
ISBN: 9798338802397
Imprint: Independently published

Cover Art: Created by the author with DALL-E

For Ebele, Añulika and Kenechi

The impact of a technology depends not only on its nature, but on how society understands and harnesses it.

Prologue

In recent years, Artificial Intelligence (AI) has moved from the realm of science fiction into reality, profoundly altering the landscape of both technology and society.

AI is set to transform how we live, work, and interact with the world around us, and, as it continues to evolve, promises to create a more connected, efficient, and personalised future. Alongside these potentially huge benefits, there are significant challenges to be overcome, with risks and dangers on a personal and global scale to be mitigated and avoided if possible.

As we stand on the cusp of this AI-driven future, it is crucial to explore, and understand, the potential directions of AI development and their impacts on multiple aspects of our lives.

Without a doubt, we are going to see some significant changes in society and our individual roles in it. The pace of AI advancement is so rapid that it is likely these changes – and societal disruption - will occur at a pace never seen before.

This book aims to provide the reader with a good understanding of AI, and what the world might look like in the not-too-distant future - delving into the likely advancements, ethical considerations, regulatory efforts, and potential societal impacts of AI. It offers a comprehensive overview of the history of AI, the current state, ongoing development and challenges, along with where this may lead us. It also features a glossary of AI terms, a list of prominent figures in the world of AI (with short biographies) and lists of current leading AI technologies.

Note from the Author

Our AI Journey is itself an exploration of the capabilities of the current state of Artificial Intelligence – the content and creation of the book is heavily supported by the latest OpenAI ChatGPT 4o tool.*

On commencing the curation of this book, I had the dual aims of deepening my high-level understanding of AI, and creating a resource that supports others who are intrigued by the topic - by providing an easy to comprehend overview, which both informs and sets in play a whole host of additional thoughts and enthusiasm for the topic.

It is my strong belief that everyone needs to be aware of what AI is and could become in the coming years – to protect themselves and others from potential dangers, maximise the benefit that AI can bring to their lives, and make decisions from an informed viewpoint. I hope that this book helps to achieve this.

Due to the pace of change in AI, it is important to note that this book is written in June to September 2024 – it is my expectation that an update/addendum will be made every 6 months (this may not be frequent enough, but let's see!).

* I have endeavoured to credit those responsible for the original thought that has inspired ChatGPT in the references section at the end of this book. Those that have used these tools will, I am sure, concur that it is currently not easy to ensure all original source material is referenced in the output. Please contact the author if you believe your original thought has not been referenced. This does not affect the copyright of this book.

About the Author

Neil Mayes has over 20 years of business experience, encompassing product development, manufacturing, B2C and B2B sales, customer service, marketing and communications. He also holds a Master's degree in Engineering (Product Design & Manufacture), an Executive MBA, and is a Certified ANA Marketing Professional.

Neil lives in London, UK, is married and has three young children. He hopes his children can grow up in a world where the deployment of AI is for the betterment of the whole population, creating a fairer and more equitable world than the present day.

Contents

Introduction to AI and the Importance of Understanding It 1

  AI in Everyday Life 1

  Why Understanding AI Matters 2

  The Future of AI 3

SECTION 1 – A HISTORY OF AI..5

  The History of AI: A Journey Through Time 5

SECTION 2 – HOT TOPICS IN AI 11

  Chapter 1: AGI (Artificial General Intelligence).................... 11

  Chapter 2: Text-to-Image and Text-to-Video Tools 16

  Chapter 3: GPTs and Large Language Models (LLMs)...... 22

  Chapter 4: Specialised GPTs and Domain-Specific AI: Tailoring AI for Specific Needs 28

  Chapter 5: Robotics and AI: From Fiction to Reality 34

SECTION 3 – CURRENT THEMES IN AI 41

  Introduction 41

  Chapter 6: Generative AI.. 41

  Chapter 7: Autonomous AI Agents 45

  Chapter 8: AI in Robotics 48

  Chapter 9: AI in the Workplace 51

  Chapter 10: Regulation and Policy...................................... 54

  Chapter 11: Responsible AI.. 57

  Chapter 12: AI Misuse and Incidents.................................. 60

  Chapter 13: Deepfakes 64

  Chapter 14: AI and Elections.. 67

  Chapter 15: Hardware and Infrastructure............................ 70

SECTION 4 – THE FUTURE OF AI AND HUMAN SOCIETY.................73

  Chapter 16: The Potential for AI to Address Key Challenges in Human Society 73

  Chapter 17: AI's Impact on Society: The Hollywood Strikes.............. 81

Chapter 18: Mitigating the Impacts of War 85

Chapter 19: Risk of Malevolent AI Including Incorporation in Robotics 87

Chapter 20: AI and Governments: Supporting the Achievement of Societal Challenges 91

Chapter 21: Constraints on Future Speed of AI Development - Challenges and Solutions..95

SECTION 5 – OUR AI TOMORROW 103

Chapter 22: Forecast - Top 10 Uses for AI in Everyday Life............ 103

Chapter 23: Scenarios for AI Development and Its Impact on Human Society Over the Next 15 Years 108

Chapter 24: The Future Human Society with AI: A 20-Year Forecast by AI 116

Chapter 25: Preparing for this Future... 135

SECTION 6 – GLOSSARY, AI INFLUENCERS & LEADING AI TOOLS 141

Glossary of Terms for All Things AI 141

Most Influential People in the AI Industry 149

Top 100 Most Significant AI Tools.. 158

Conversational AI Agents 166

Customer Service and Support AI Agents 167

Virtual Personal Assistants... 168

AI Agents for Business and Productivity... 169

Specialised AI Agents... 170

AI Agents for Autonomous Systems 171

AI Agents in Healthcare.. 172

AI Agents for Finance... 173

Miscellaneous AI Agents 174

AI Agents for Personal Use 175

AI Agents for Entertainment 176

REFERENCES 178

Introduction to AI and the Importance of Understanding It

Artificial Intelligence (AI) is a term that has increasingly become part of our everyday conversations, from news headlines to casual discussions about the latest tech gadgets. But what exactly is AI, and why is it important for everyone to understand it?

AI refers to the simulation of human intelligence in machines that are designed to think and act like humans. These intelligent systems can perform tasks that typically require human intelligence, such as learning, reasoning, problem-solving, perception, and language understanding. The applications of AI are vast and varied, impacting numerous aspects of our lives, from the way we communicate and work, to how we shop and entertain ourselves.

AI in Everyday Life

AI is all around us, often in ways we might not even notice. Voice-activated assistants, like Siri and Alexa, use AI to understand and respond to our questions. Streaming services, such as Netflix and Spotify, use AI to recommend shows and music based on our preferences. Even the ads we see online are often curated by AI algorithms designed to target us with products we're more likely to be interested in.

In healthcare, AI aids doctors in diagnosing diseases and personalising treatment plans. In finance, AI helps detect fraudulent activities and manage investment portfolios. In education, AI-powered tools provide personalised learning experiences for students.

The reach of AI now extends to almost every sector of industry, making it a crucial part of modern society – this is only going to deepen over the coming years.

Why Understanding AI Matters

Understanding AI is, and will become ever more, essential for several reasons: -

Empowerment Through Knowledge:

By understanding how AI works, individuals can make informed decisions about the technologies they use, careers they pursue, and skills they seek to learn. This knowledge helps people choose products and services that best meet their needs, and make decisions that are more likely to withstand the continued expansion of AI.

Enhanced Job Prospects:

As AI continues to transform the job market, having a basic understanding of AI can open new career opportunities and help individuals stay relevant in their fields. Whether you're a healthcare professional, educator, or engineer, knowing how AI can augment your work is increasingly important.

Ethical Awareness:

AI technologies raise significant ethical questions about privacy, security, and bias. Understanding AI enables people to critically evaluate these issues and advocate for responsible AI development and deployment.

Digital Literacy:

In a world where digital skills are becoming as essential as reading and writing, AI literacy is a crucial component. Understanding AI helps individuals navigate the digital landscape more effectively, from social media to online shopping.

Civic Engagement:

AI is shaping public policy and governance in profound ways. An informed public can engage better in discussions about AI regulation, ethical standards, and its societal impact, ensuring that AI technologies are developed and used in ways that benefit everyone.

Preparing Children for the Future

As AI increasingly shapes the world we live in, preparing children for an AI-driven future is essential to ensure they thrive in a rapidly changing society: By teaching them future-ready skills like critical thinking, creativity, and emotional intelligence, we can prepare them for roles that AI cannot easily replicate.

The Future of AI

Looking ahead, AI holds the promise of solving some of humanity's most pressing challenges. It has the potential to revolutionise healthcare by enabling early disease detection and personalised treatments. It can help combat climate change by optimising energy use, enhancing carbon capture technologies, and monitoring environmental changes. AI can also enhance education by providing tailored learning experiences and supporting teachers in the classroom.

However, the rapid advancement of AI also comes with risks and challenges. Issues such as job displacement, privacy concerns, and the potential misuse of AI technologies, need to be addressed through thoughtful regulation and ethical practices.

Artificial Intelligence is not just a technological breakthrough; it is a transformative force that is reshaping our world. Understanding AI is crucial for navigating this new landscape and making informed decisions, therefore, as AI continues to evolve, it is essential for everyone to stay informed and engaged with its development and implications. This knowledge will empower us to harness the benefits of AI while mitigating its risks, creating a better and more equitable future for all.

SECTION 1 – A HISTORY OF AI

The History of AI: A Journey Through Time

Artificial Intelligence has a fascinating history spanning several decades, marked by groundbreaking achievements and milestones that have shaped the technology into what it is today. This section explores the evolution of AI, from its conceptual beginnings to the sophisticated systems we encounter in our daily lives today.

Early Beginnings and Conceptual Foundations

The idea of intelligent machines dates back to ancient times, with myths and stories featuring automatons and mechanical beings. However, the conceptual foundation of AI really began in the mid-20th century with the advent of computer science and formal logic.

Alan Turing and the Turing Test (1950)

Alan Turing, a British mathematician, is often considered the father of computer science and AI. In 1950, he published a seminal paper titled "Computing Machinery and Intelligence," in which he proposed the idea of a machine that could simulate any human intelligence task. Turing introduced the 'Turing Test', a criterion for determining whether a machine can exhibit intelligent behaviour indistinguishable from that of a human.

The Turing Test continues to serve as a foundational benchmark in evaluating artificial intelligence, assessing whether a machine's behaviour can indistinguishably mimic human responses, thus stimulating ongoing advancements and discussions in the field of AI research.

The Dartmouth Conference (1956)

The Dartmouth Conference, held in the summer of 1956, is widely regarded as the birth of AI as a field of study. Organised by John McCarthy, Marvin Minsky, Nathaniel Rochester, and Claude Shannon, this conference brought together leading researchers to discuss the possibility of creating intelligent machines. The term "Artificial Intelligence" was coined during this conference, marking the formal establishment of AI as a scientific discipline.

The Early Years: Symbolic AI and Rule-Based Systems

The initial decades of AI research were characterised by the development of symbolic AI, which focused on using symbols and rules to represent and manipulate knowledge – 'Symbolic Logic'.

The Logic Theorist (1956)

Developed by Allen Newell and Herbert A. Simon, the Logic Theorist was one of the first AI programmes. It was designed to mimic human problem-solving by using symbolic logic to prove mathematical theorems. This pioneering work demonstrated the potential of AI to perform tasks that required reasoning and symbolic manipulation.

ELIZA (1966)

Joseph Weizenbaum created ELIZA, an early natural language processing programme that could simulate conversation with a human by using pattern matching and substitution techniques. ELIZA's ability to engage in seemingly meaningful dialogue with users highlighted the potential of AI in understanding and generating human language.

The Rise of Machine Learning and Neural Networks

While symbolic AI made significant strides, researchers soon realised the limitations of rule-based systems (e.g. lack of scalability, flexibility and adaptability). This led to the exploration of machine learning and neural networks, inspired by the human brain's structure and learning processes.

Perceptron (1957)

Frank Rosenblatt developed the Perceptron, an early type of artificial neural network. The Perceptron was capable of learning from data and making simple classifications, laying the groundwork for more complex neural networks.

Backpropagation and Neural Networks Revival (1986)

The 1980s saw a resurgence of interest in neural networks, particularly with the development of the backpropagation algorithm* by David Rumelhart, Geoffrey Hinton, and Ronald Williams. This algorithm allowed multi-layer neural networks to learn from data more effectively, enabling the development of more sophisticated AI models. Backpropagation became a cornerstone of modern deep learning techniques.

*Backpropagation is like a teacher grading a test and then helping a student learn from their mistakes so they can do better next time.

The Advent of Deep Learning and Big Data

The 21st century ushered in the era of big data and deep learning, revolutionising AI with the ability to process vast amounts of data and extract meaningful patterns.

ImageNet and AlexNet (2012)

The ImageNet project, led by Fei-Fei Li, provided a large-scale dataset of labelled images, which became a benchmark for evaluating computer vision algorithms. In 2012, AlexNet, a deep convolutional neural network (CNN – see glossary) developed by Alex Krizhevsky, Ilya Sutskever, and Geoffrey Hinton, achieved a groundbreaking performance in the ImageNet competition/test. This achievement demonstrated the power of deep learning and sparked a wave of advancements, key developments, and milestones in deep learning and artificial intelligence – including the development of Generative Models (GANs) and Natural Language Processing (NLP).

AlphaGo (2016)

AlphaGo, developed by DeepMind, made headlines when it defeated the world champion Go player Lee Sedol in 2016. Go, a complex board game with more possible moves than there are atoms in the universe, was long considered a grand challenge for AI. AlphaGo's success, achieved through a combination of deep learning and reinforcement learning, showcased the remarkable potential of AI to master tasks requiring strategic thinking and intuition.

Recent Advancements and the Future of AI

In recent years, AI has continued to advance at a rapid pace, with significant developments in various fields, from natural language processing to autonomous systems.

GPT-3 and Natural Language Processing (2020)

OpenAI's GPT-3 (Generative Pre-trained Transformer 3) set a new standard for natural language processing with its ability to generate human-like text based on context. With 175 billion parameters, GPT-3 can perform a wide range of language tasks, including translation, summarisation, and content generation. Its capabilities have opened up new possibilities for AI applications in communication, education, and creative industries.

Autonomous Vehicles and AI in Robotics

Autonomous vehicles, powered by AI, are poised to transform transportation. Companies like Tesla, Waymo, and Uber are developing self-driving cars that use AI to navigate complex environments, make real-time decisions, and improve road safety. Similarly, AI in robotics is advancing rapidly, with applications ranging from industrial automation to healthcare, where robots assist in surgeries and provide care to patients.

Conclusion

The journey of AI from its conceptual beginnings to the present day is a story of relentless human innovation and discovery. Key milestones and achievements have marked significant progress, transforming AI from a theoretical concept into a practical and impactful technology. As AI continues to evolve, it holds the promise of driving further advancements and shaping the future of human society in ways we are only beginning to imagine.

SECTION 2 – HOT TOPICS IN AI

Chapter 1: AGI (Artificial General Intelligence)

One of the first terms you may hear banded around in AI conversations is 'AGI'. This stands for 'Artificial General Intelligence' and refers to a level of artificial intelligence that can understand, learn, and apply knowledge across a wide range of tasks, mirroring the cognitive abilities of a human being.

Unlike other AI, which is often designed to perform specific tasks, AGI possesses the versatility and adaptability to handle various activities and solve problems in different domains without requiring specialised programming for each task. AGI is often depicted as the ultimate goal in the field of AI research, representing a machine with the ability to perform any intellectual task that a human can.

Key Characteristics of AGI

AGI possesses a range of advanced capabilities that enable it to understand, learn, and apply knowledge across diverse domains. The key characteristics that define AGI are:

>*Generalisation:* AGI can generalise knowledge from one domain to another, applying learned concepts to new and unfamiliar situations. This ability to transfer knowledge and skills across different contexts distinguishes AGI from narrow AI.

>*Adaptability:* AGI can adapt to new environments and challenges without human intervention. It can learn from its

experiences and modify its behaviour to improve performance in a wide range of tasks.

Autonomy: AGI operates autonomously, making decisions and taking actions independently. It does not rely on pre-defined rules or specific programming to function effectively.

Human-Like Cognitive Abilities: AGI exhibits cognitive abilities similar to those of humans, including reasoning, problem-solving, perception, language understanding, and creativity. It can engage in abstract thinking and comprehend complex concepts.

Potential Benefits of AGI

The advent of Artificial General Intelligence (AGI) holds the promise of revolutionising numerous aspects of human life. With its ability to understand, learn, and apply knowledge across various domains, AGI could offer unprecedented benefits that extend far beyond the capabilities of current AI systems. Some of the potential benefits of AGI include:

Problem-Solving: AGI could solve complex global challenges, such as climate change, disease eradication, and resource management. Its ability to analyse vast amounts of data and generate innovative solutions could lead to breakthroughs in various fields.

Automation and Efficiency: AGI could automate a wide range of tasks across industries, increasing efficiency and productivity. This could lead to significant economic growth and improved quality of life.

Personalised Services: AGI could provide highly personalised services in healthcare, education, and entertainment. It could tailor treatments, learning experiences, and content to individual needs and preferences.

Scientific Advancements: AGI could accelerate scientific research by conducting experiments, analysing data, and generating hypotheses. It could assist researchers in making new discoveries and advancing human knowledge.

Challenges and Risks

While the potential benefits of Artificial General Intelligence (AGI) are immense, its development also brings significant challenges and risks that must be carefully managed. As we move closer to realising AGI, it is crucial to address these concerns to ensure that its impact on society is positive and sustainable. The following are some of the primary challenges and risks associated with AGI:

Ethical Concerns: The development of AGI raises ethical questions about its use, control, and impact on society. Ensuring that AGI is aligned with human values and operates ethically is a significant challenge.

Safety and Control: AGI's autonomy and decision-making capabilities pose risks if not properly controlled. There is a need for robust safety mechanisms to prevent unintended consequences and ensure that AGI acts in the best interest of humanity.

Economic Disruption: The widespread adoption of AGI could lead to job displacement and economic inequality. Addressing these potential disruptions requires thoughtful planning and policy interventions.

Existential Risk: Some experts argue that AGI could pose an existential risk if it surpasses human intelligence and becomes uncontrollable. Ensuring that AGI remains aligned with human goals is crucial to mitigating this risk.

Current State of AGI Research

While significant progress has been made in AI research, achieving AGI remains a relatively distant goal (although some leading figures in AI claim that we may see this during 2025!). Current AI systems, including advanced machine learning models and deep neural networks, are still limited to narrow applications. Researchers are exploring various approaches to develop AGI, including:

Neuroscience-Inspired Models: Studying the human brain and its cognitive processes to develop AI systems that mimic human intelligence.

Hybrid Approaches: Combining symbolic AI (which uses explicit rules and logic) with machine learning to create more flexible and generalisable AI systems.

Transfer Learning: Developing methods that enable AI systems to transfer knowledge from one domain to another, enhancing their generalisation capabilities.

Reinforcement Learning: Using reinforcement learning techniques to train AI systems to learn from their interactions with the environment and improve their performance over time.

Conclusion

Artificial General Intelligence would represent a transformative milestone in the field of AI, with the potential to revolutionise multiple aspects of human life. While the benefits of AGI could be immense, so are the challenges and risks associated with its development. Ensuring that AGI is developed and deployed responsibly, ethically, and safely is paramount to realising its potential while safeguarding humanity's future. As research progresses, ongoing dialogue and collaboration among scientists, policymakers, ethicists, and the public will be essential in navigating the complex landscape of AGI.

Chapter 2: Text-to-Image and Text-to-Video Tools

The advent of text-to-image and text-to-video tools in recent years represents a significant leap forward in AI capabilities (and they continue to develop at a great pace), allowing users to generate visual content from text descriptions. These tools leverage advanced deep learning models, particularly Generative Adversarial Networks (GANs) and Transformers, to interpret and visualise text inputs. This chapter explores the functionality, interaction methods, and ongoing development of these tools.

Interaction and Capabilities

These text-to-image and text-to-video tools provide users with a range of interaction methods, from simple web interfaces and APIs to more sophisticated drag-and-drop and collaborative platforms. Their capabilities span from generating realistic and artistic images, to creating professional-quality videos with AI avatars and automated voiceovers.

Ongoing Development

The ongoing development in this field focuses on several key areas:

Quality and Realism: Enhancing the resolution, detail, and realism of generated images and videos.

User Experience: Improving user interfaces and interaction methods to make these tools more accessible and intuitive.

Customisation: Offering more customisation options for users to tailor the generated content to their specific needs.

Ethical Considerations: Addressing issues related to bias, misuse, and ethical implications of generated content.

Popular Text-to-Image Tools

At the time of writing the following represent some of the most popular Text-to-Image tools:

DALL-E (OpenAI)

- o **Interaction**: Users can input detailed textual descriptions through a web interface or API to generate images.
- o **Capabilities**: DALL-E can create highly detailed and diverse images from textual descriptions, including abstract and imaginative concepts.
- o **Ongoing Development**: Continual improvements in understanding and rendering complex descriptions, increasing the resolution and quality of generated images.

MidJourney

- o **Interaction**: Accessible via a web interface and Discord bot, allowing users to input text prompts and receive generated images.

- Capabilities: Specialises in artistic and surreal image generation, providing users with visually striking interpretations of their descriptions.

- Ongoing Development: Enhancing the artistic style and variety of generated images, expanding user interaction features.

DeepArt.io

- Interaction: Users upload an image and provide a style reference to generate new images in that style, combined with their textual inputs.

- Capabilities: Transforms photos into artworks using styles from famous paintings, leveraging neural style transfer techniques.

- Ongoing Development: Improving the accuracy and quality of style transfer, integrating more artistic styles and user controls.

Artbreeder

- Interaction: Users can manipulate images through a combination of text inputs and interactive sliders, blending multiple images and styles.

- Capabilities: Generates and morphs images based on genetic algorithms, allowing collaborative creation and refinement.

- Ongoing Development: Enhancing user collaboration features and expanding the range of image styles and genetic traits.

Runway ML

- o **Interaction**: Provides a user-friendly interface for generating images from text, also offers API access for developers.

- o **Capabilities**: Supports various generative models, including StyleGAN and BigGAN, for creating realistic and artistic images.

- o **Ongoing Development**: Integrating more generative models and improving the usability and flexibility of the interface.

Popular Text-to-Video Tools

At the time of writing the following some of the most popular Text-to-Video tools:

Synthesia

- o **Interaction**: Users can create videos by inputting text scripts, choosing avatars, and selecting voiceovers through a web platform.

- o **Capabilities**: Generates professional-looking videos with AI avatars that lip-sync to the input text, ideal for business and educational content.

- o **Ongoing Development**: Adding more avatars, languages, and customisation options, improving lip-sync accuracy and video quality.

Pictory

- ○ **Interaction**: Users can input text summaries or scripts, and the tool generates video summaries with relevant visuals and voiceovers.

- ○ **Capabilities**: Automates video creation from articles and blog posts, providing a quick way to generate engaging video content.

- ○ **Ongoing Development**: Enhancing visual and audio quality, integrating more visual styles and voice options.

Lumen5

- ○ **Interaction**: Converts text content into video using a drag-and-drop interface, allowing users to customise visuals and music.

- ○ **Capabilities**: Focuses on creating social media-friendly videos from blog posts, news articles, and other textual content.

- ○ **Ongoing Development**: Expanding the library of visual assets and templates, improving text-to-video conversion accuracy.

DeepBrain

- ○ **Interaction**: Users provide text scripts, which the tool converts into videos with AI-generated presenters and backgrounds.

- Capabilities: Suitable for creating explainer videos, presentations, and educational content with virtual hosts.
- Ongoing Development: Increasing the diversity of AI presenters and backgrounds, enhancing natural language processing for more accurate script interpretation.

Animoto

- Interaction: Allows users to create videos from text and image inputs using a simple drag-and-drop interface.
- Capabilities: Offers a range of templates and customisation options to produce professional-quality videos for marketing, education, and social media.
- Ongoing Development: Improving template variety and customisation features, integrating AI-driven suggestions for video enhancements.

Conclusion

The landscape of text-to-image and text-to-video tools is rapidly evolving, driven by advances in AI and user demand for more creative and automated content generation solutions. These tools empower users to visualise their ideas and create engaging content with minimal technical expertise, heralding a new era of digital creativity and productivity. (You can see some examples of DALL-E in action later in the book.)

Our AI Journey

Chapter 3: GPTs and Large Language Models (LLMs)

You may have already encountered mention of GPTs (Generative Pre-trained Transformers) in the mainstream news (as well as earlier in this book)- these are a specific type of LLM developed by OpenAI.

Large Language Models (LLMs) are sophisticated artificial intelligence systems designed to process, understand, and generate human language. They leverage deep learning, particularly transformer architectures, to analyse vast amounts of text data, capturing linguistic nuances and contextual meanings. LLMs have significantly advanced the field of natural language processing (NLP), enabling various applications that were previously thought unattainable.

Key Characteristics of LLMs

The following key characteristics distinguish LLMs and enable their impressive capabilities across various applications:

> *Scale and Complexity:* LLMs are distinguished by their enormous scale, often consisting of billions to trillions of parameters. This extensive scale allows them to learn intricate patterns and relationships within the language.

> *Pre-training and Fine-tuning:* These models undergo a two-step training process. First, they are pre-trained on a large and diverse dataset, which enables them to learn general language features. Then, they are fine-tuned on specific tasks or domains to improve their performance on particular applications.

Contextual Understanding: LLMs can maintain context over long passages of text, allowing them to generate coherent and relevant responses. This capability is essential for tasks like conversational agents and content creation.

Versatility: LLMs are capable of performing a wide range of NLP tasks, including text generation, translation, summarisation, sentiment analysis, and question-answering.

Relationship Between LLMs and GPTs

The GPT architecture has become synonymous with advanced language models due to its groundbreaking capabilities and wide-ranging applications. Here's how GPTs fit into the broader category of LLMs:

Transformers Architecture: GPTs are built on the transformer architecture, which utilises self-attention mechanisms to handle long-range dependencies in text. This architecture has been pivotal in the success of GPT models and other LLMs.

Generative Capabilities: As their name suggests, GPTs are particularly focused on generative tasks. They excel at generating human-like text, making them useful for applications such as chatbots, automated content creation, and creative writing – like some sections of this book!

Pre-training and Fine-tuning: GPT models follow the standard two-step process of LLMs—pre-training on a vast amount of text followed by fine-tuning on specific datasets. This process allows GPTs to achieve state-of-the-art performance across various NLP tasks.

Versions and Improvements: Since the release of GPT-2, each subsequent version (e.g., GPT-3, GPT-4) has seen significant improvements in scale, performance, and versatility. These enhancements have expanded the range of applications, and the quality of outputs generated by GPT models.

Potential Benefits of LLMs and GPTs

These models offer a range of benefits that have the potential to transform various industries and aspects of daily life including:

Enhanced Communication: LLMs and GPTs improve human-computer interaction through more natural and intuitive communication in applications like virtual assistants and customer service chatbots.

Content Generation: These models can generate high-quality text content, such as articles, reports, and creative works, thereby supporting various industries like journalism, marketing, and entertainment.

Language Translation: LLMs and GPTs can provide accurate, context-aware translations, facilitating global communication and collaboration.

Educational Tools: They can assist in personalised learning by providing tailored explanations, tutoring, and feedback to students, as well as creating educational content and resources.

Challenges and Risks

While LLMs and GPTs offer significant benefits, their development and deployment are accompanied by several challenges and risks that need to be carefully managed. Addressing these issues is essential to ensure that these powerful AI tools are used responsibly and ethically. The key challenges and risks associated with LLMs and GPTs include:

Bias and Fairness: LLMs and GPTs can inherit and amplify biases present in their training data, leading to unfair or discriminatory outcomes. Addressing these biases is crucial to ensure fair and ethical AI use.

Misinformation and Manipulation: These models can generate realistic but false information, posing risks of misinformation and malicious use, such as creating deepfake content.

Privacy Concerns: LLMs trained on large datasets may inadvertently learn and reproduce sensitive or private information. Ensuring data privacy and security is essential.

Ethical Use: The powerful capabilities of LLMs and GPTs necessitate ethical guidelines and frameworks to prevent misuse and ensure responsible deployment.

Current State of LLM and GPT Research

Research in LLMs and GPTs is rapidly evolving, driven by the continuous advancements in AI and deep learning technologies. Key areas of focus include:

> *Model Scaling:* Researchers are exploring ways to scale models even further, aiming for higher performance and more nuanced language understanding.

> *Efficiency Improvements*: Efforts are being made to improve the computational efficiency of these models, reducing the resources required for training and inference.

> *Bias Mitigation:* Techniques to detect and mitigate biases in LLMs and GPTs are being developed to ensure fair and unbiased AI systems.

> *Ethical and Safe AI:* Ongoing work aims to establish robust ethical standards and safety measures for deploying LLMs and GPTs, ensuring their benefits are maximised while minimising risks.

Conclusion

Large Language Models, particularly GPTs, represent a significant leap forward in the capabilities of AI to understand and generate human language. Their versatility, contextual understanding, and generative capabilities open up numerous possibilities across various domains. However, the challenges and risks associated with these powerful models must be addressed through continued research, ethical guidelines, and responsible deployment practices. As LLMs and GPTs continue to evolve, they hold the promise of transforming how we interact with technology and each other, heralding a new era in artificial intelligence.

Chapter 4: Specialised GPTs and Domain-Specific AI: Tailoring AI for Specific Needs

The advent of specialised Generative Pre-trained Transformers (GPTs) and domain-specific AI marks a significant evolution in artificial intelligence. These tailored AI systems are designed to excel in particular fields, offering unprecedented accuracy, efficiency, and relevance. This section delves into the development and application of specialised GPTs, their impact on various industries, and how domain-specific training is driving AI to new heights.

The Evolution of Specialised GPTs

Generative Pre-trained Transformers (GPTs) have revolutionised natural language processing (NLP), with models like GPT-4o and Claude demonstrating remarkable abilities in understanding and generating human-like text.

General-purpose GPTs are trained on diverse datasets encompassing a wide range of topics. This broad training enables them to handle various tasks but can sometimes result in less precise outputs for niche areas. In contrast, specialised GPTs are fine-tuned on domain-specific data, allowing them to achieve higher accuracy and relevance in their particular fields.

The Rise of Domain-Specific AI

The need for domain-specific AI arises from the unique requirements of different industries. For instance, legal professionals, medical practitioners, financial analysts, and educators each have distinct needs that a generalised AI might not address adequately. By training AI models on specialised datasets, we can create AI systems that understand the nuances and complexities of specific domains.

Enhancing AI Capabilities through Domain-Specific Training

The success of specialised GPTs hinges on the quality and relevance of the training data. By leveraging domain-specific datasets, AI models can achieve a deeper understanding of particular fields, resulting in more accurate and contextually appropriate outputs. Due to the multi-lingual nature of AI, it can also be trained on research papers/data from almost any global source – this radically enhances the breadth and depth of information available to the domain-specific AI enhancing its knowledgebase beyond the capabilities of almost any human.

The Importance of Curated Training Data

Curating high-quality, domain-specific training data is crucial for developing effective specialised GPTs. This data must be comprehensive, up-to-date, and representative of the domain's intricacies. For instance, training a medical GPT requires access to the latest clinical research, patient records, and treatment guidelines, ensuring the model's recommendations are based on the most current knowledge.

Continuous Learning and Adaptation

To maintain their relevance, specialised GPTs must undergo continuous learning and adaptation. This involves regularly updating the training data to reflect new developments, trends, and discoveries within the domain. For example, a legal GPT must be updated with new laws, court rulings, and legal precedents to provide accurate and current information to legal professionals.

Addressing Ethical and Privacy Concerns

Developing specialised GPTs also involves addressing ethical and privacy concerns, particularly when handling sensitive data. Ensuring data privacy, obtaining informed consent, and implementing robust security measures are essential to maintain trust and integrity. In healthcare, for instance, specialised GPTs must comply with regulations such as HIPAA (Health Insurance Portability and Accountability Act) to protect patient confidentiality.

Driving Innovation with Specialised AI

The integration of specialised GPTs into various industries is driving innovation and unlocking new possibilities. These AI systems are not only enhancing existing processes but also enabling the development of novel applications that were previously unimaginable.

Achievements and Applications of Specialised GPTs

The development and deployment of specialised GPTs has led to significant advancements across various sectors. These tailored AI systems are transforming industries by providing expert-level assistance, improving efficiency, and enabling innovative applications.

GPT-3 for Legal Research

In the legal field, specialised GPTs have been trained on extensive legal texts, including statutes, case law, and legal commentary. These models assist lawyers in conducting legal research, drafting documents, and analysing case details with remarkable accuracy. For example, Casetext's AI tool, "CoCounsel," leverages a specialised GPT to provide legal professionals with precise and relevant information, significantly reducing the time and effort required for research.

Medical GPTs for Healthcare

The healthcare industry has benefited immensely from specialised GPTs trained on medical literature, clinical guidelines, and patient records. These AI models assist doctors in diagnosing diseases, recommending treatments, and keeping up with the latest medical research. IBM's Watson for Oncology, for instance, uses specialised AI to analyse vast amounts of medical data, helping oncologists develop personalised treatment plans for cancer patients.

Financial Analysis with AI

In the financial sector, specialised GPTs are trained on financial reports, market data, and economic indicators. These models can perform complex financial analysis, predict market trends, and generate detailed reports. BloombergGPT, for example, is designed to assist financial analysts by providing accurate and timely insights into market movements and economic developments.

AI in Education: Personalised Learning

In education, specialised GPTs are being used to create personalised learning experiences. By analysing students' learning styles, strengths, and weaknesses, AI models can tailor educational content to meet individual needs. For example, AI-powered tutoring systems can provide customised exercises and feedback, helping students master complex subjects at their own pace.

AI in Creative Industries: Enhanced Creativity

Specialised GPTs are also making their mark in creative industries, assisting artists, writers, and designers in their work. These AI models can generate ideas, provide inspiration, and even create original content. For instance, Jukedeck, an AI music composition tool, uses specialised algorithms to compose music based on user inputs, enabling musicians to explore new creative directions.

AI in Customer Service: Improved Interaction

In customer service, specialised GPTs enhance interaction by providing accurate and contextually relevant responses to customer inquiries. AI-powered chatbots and virtual assistants can handle a wide range of customer service tasks, from answering FAQs to resolving complex issues. Companies like Zendesk and LivePerson leverage specialised AI to improve customer satisfaction and operational efficiency.

Conclusion

The development of specialised GPTs and domain-specific AI represents another big leap forward in artificial intelligence. By tailoring AI systems to excel in particular areas, we can achieve higher accuracy, efficiency, and relevance, transforming industries and enhancing human capabilities on a global basis.

As we continue to refine and expand these specialised models, the potential applications are limitless, promising a future where AI seamlessly integrates into every facet of our lives, providing expert assistance and driving innovation.

Chapter 5: Robotics and AI: From Fiction to Reality

Robotics and AI have evolved hand-in-hand over the decades, transforming the realm of science fiction into tangible reality. This section explores the historical development of robotics, significant milestones and achievements, and the ways AI is enhancing robotic capabilities through simulated real-world training.

Asimov's Laws of Robotics

Before we dive into the history and advancements, it's essential to touch upon Isaac Asimov's laws of robotics, which have profoundly influenced both the ethical framework and popular imagination surrounding robotics. Introduced in Asimov's 1942 short story "Runaround," the Three Laws of Robotics are:

1. **A robot may not injure a human being or, through inaction, allow a human being to come to harm.**

2. **A robot must obey the orders given it by human beings except where such orders would conflict with the First Law.**

3. **A robot must protect its own existence as long as such protection does not conflict with the First or Second Law.**

These laws were designed to ensure the safety and ethical use of robots, anticipating many of the real-world concerns that arise as we integrate AI and robotics into daily life.

While Asimov's Three Laws of Robotics are not directly implemented in current AI systems, they continue to influence the ethical and philosophical discussion surrounding AI development. Modern AI research and development prioritise safety, ethical behaviour, and human well-being, aligning with the spirit of Asimov's vision. However, the complexity of real-world AI applications requires more nuanced and technically feasible approaches than the straightforward laws proposed in science fiction.

Early Developments and Milestones

The journey of robotics began long before the term "robot" was coined. Early mechanical automatons, such as those created by the Greek engineer Hero of Alexandria, laid the groundwork for future innovations. However, the modern era of robotics truly began in the 20th century.

The Birth of the Modern Robot: Unimate (1961)

The first industrial robot, Unimate, was introduced by George Devol and Joseph Engelberger. Installed in a General Motors plant in 1961, Unimate performed repetitive tasks such as welding and material handling. This marked the beginning of robotics in manufacturing, revolutionising production lines and increasing efficiency.

The Stanford Arm (1969)

Developed by Victor Scheinman at Stanford University, the Stanford Arm was one of the first electrically powered, computer-controlled robotic arms. It featured six degrees of freedom ('ranges of movement'), allowing it to perform a variety of complex tasks. The Stanford Arm set the stage for future advancements in robotic manipulation and control.

Shakey the Robot (1966-1972)

Shakey, developed at the Stanford Research Institute (SRI), was the first robot capable of reasoning about its actions. Equipped with sensors, cameras, and a computer, Shakey could navigate its environment, plan tasks, and avoid obstacles. This project was a stride towards integrating AI with robotics, demonstrating the potential for autonomous decision-making.

The Rise of AI in Robotics

As AI technologies have advanced, their integration with robotics has led to significant enhancements in robot capabilities. Machine learning, computer vision, and natural language processing have all contributed to the development of more intelligent and adaptable robots.

The Development of ASIMO (2000)

ASIMO, created by Honda, is one of the most famous humanoid robots. Unveiled in 2000, ASIMO could walk, run, climb stairs, and interact with people. It represented a significant achievement in robotics, showcasing advanced mobility and human-robot interaction capabilities. ASIMO's development involved extensive research in biomechanics, control systems, and AI, making it a symbol of robotic potential.

Boston Dynamics and the Evolution of Dynamic Robots

Boston Dynamics has been at the forefront of developing dynamic robots capable of navigating complex environments.

Robots like BigDog, Spot, and Atlas have demonstrated remarkable agility, balance, and adaptability. For example, Atlas can perform backflips, navigate uneven terrain, and even dance. These robots are equipped with sophisticated sensors and AI algorithms that enable real-time decision-making and adaptation.

Robotic Surgery: da Vinci Surgical System

The da Vinci Surgical System, developed by Intuitive Surgical, revolutionised minimally invasive surgery. Introduced in the early 2000s, this robotic system allows surgeons to perform delicate procedures with greater precision and control. The integration of AI helps in enhancing the system's capabilities, providing real-time feedback and guidance to surgeons.

Enhancing Robot Capabilities with AI and Simulated Real-World Training

One of the most transformative advancements in robotics has been the use of AI to simulate real-world training environments. By leveraging large-scale simulations, robots can be trained to handle a multitude of scenarios, improving their performance and adaptability.

Simulated Training with AI: The Role of Reinforcement Learning

Reinforcement learning, a type of machine learning, has become a crucial tool for training robots. In this approach, robots learn by interacting with their environment and receiving feedback in the form of rewards or penalties. Simulations provide a safe and scalable way to expose robots to thousands of different scenarios, allowing them to learn and adapt without the risks associated with physical trials.

OpenAI's Dactyl: Mastering Rubik's Cube with Simulated Training

OpenAI's Dactyl project is a prime example of using simulated training to enhance robotic capabilities. Dactyl, a robotic hand, was trained in a simulated environment to manipulate a Rubik's Cube. By practicing in thousands of simulated scenarios, the AI behind Dactyl learned to handle the cube with remarkable dexterity and precision. This project demonstrated the power of simulation in achieving complex motor skills that are challenging to replicate in the physical world.

Autonomous Vehicles: Learning through Simulation

Autonomous vehicles rely heavily on AI and simulated training to navigate real-world environments. Companies like Waymo and Tesla use sophisticated simulations to train their self-driving cars, exposing them to countless driving scenarios, from busy urban streets to rural highways. These simulations help the AI systems learn to recognise and respond to a wide variety of situations, enhancing safety and reliability on the road.

Sim2Real Transfer: Bridging the Gap between Simulation and Reality

One of the critical challenges in simulated training is the Sim2Real transfer, which involves ensuring that skills learned in simulation can be effectively applied in the real world. Researchers use techniques like domain randomisation, which varies the simulation parameters to teach robots to handle a broad range of real-world conditions. This approach has been successful in training robots for tasks like object recognition, manipulation, and autonomous navigation.

The Future of Robotics and AI

As robotics and AI continue to advance, the integration of simulated training and real-world applications will drive the next wave of innovation. Future robots will be more intelligent, adaptable, and capable of performing complex tasks with minimal human intervention. Key areas of development include:

Collaborative Robots (Cobots)

Cobots are designed to work alongside humans, enhancing productivity and safety in various industries. They can assist with tasks that require precision, strength, or repetitive motion, while AI ensures they operate safely and efficiently alongside human workers.

AI in Healthcare Robotics

AI-powered robots will play an increasingly important role in healthcare, from assisting in surgeries to providing care for the elderly. These robots can help address workforce shortages, improve patient outcomes, and reduce healthcare costs.

Exploration and Beyond

Robotics and AI are set to revolutionise space exploration, underwater research, and hazardous environment operations. Robots equipped with AI can perform tasks that are too dangerous or impractical for humans, expanding our ability to explore and understand the world around us.

Conclusion

The history of robotics and AI is a testament to human ingenuity and the relentless pursuit of innovation. From the early automatons to today's sophisticated AI-powered robots, each milestone represents a step forward in our ability to create machines that can learn, adapt, and perform tasks autonomously. As we continue to integrate AI with robotics, the possibilities are limitless, promising a future where intelligent machines enhance our capabilities and improve our quality of life.

SECTION 3 – CURRENT THEMES IN AI

Introduction

Artificial Intelligence has continued to evolve at an unprecedented pace in 2024, influencing multiple aspects of technology and society. The top AI stories of the year highlight significant advancements, ethical considerations, regulatory developments, and the integration of AI across diverse fields. From generative AI transforming creative industries to responsible AI addressing ethical concerns, the landscape is rich with innovation and challenges.

This section delves into the key themes currently shaping AI discussions, identifying both potential positive and negative implications, providing some examples to enhance the explanation of the topic, and provide hints to the reader as to where additional study could branch from.

Chapter 6: Generative AI

Current State

Generative AI has seen remarkable progress in recent years, with sophisticated models capable of creating text, music, and multimedia content. Platforms like ElevenLabs and Suno have revolutionised content creation by automating audio and music production. ElevenLabs, valued at $1.1 billion, offers advanced voice cloning technology, while Suno transforms text prompts into complete songs. Speechify and Natural Readers meanwhile convert text into various voices, enhancing accessibility and engagement. These tools, along with text-to-image, text-to-video and GPTs (described in prior chapters), democratise creativity, enabling individuals without technical expertise to generate professional-quality content.

Future Expectations

The future of generative AI is expected to bring even more advanced models capable of producing higher quality and more diverse content. AI-generated movies, complex interactive experiences, and personalised media tailored to individual preferences are likely developments. As generative AI becomes more sophisticated, it will be able to create content that is indistinguishable from human-created works, further blurring the lines between human and machine creativity.

Positive Implications

1. *Democratisation of Creativity:* Generative AI allows anyone, regardless of their technical skills, to create high-quality content. This democratises access to creative tools and could lead to a surge in creative output across various media.

2. *Enhanced Productivity:* By automating routine creative tasks, generative AI can free up time for human creators to focus on more complex and innovative aspects of their work.

3. *Increased Accessibility:* Tools like Speechify and Natural Readers make content more accessible to people with disabilities, such as those with visual impairments, by converting text into audio.

Negative Implications

1. *Job Displacement:* As AI takes over more creative tasks, there is a risk that jobs in creative industries could be lost, particularly those that involve routine or repetitive work.

2. *Intellectual Property Issues:* The widespread use of AI-generated content raises questions about ownership and intellectual property rights. Determining who owns the rights to AI-generated works could become increasingly complex.

3. *Ethical Concerns:* There is a risk that generative AI could be used to create misleading or harmful content, such as deepfakes or propaganda, which could have serious societal implications.

Examples

ElevenLabs: Imagine a podcaster who, instead of spending hours recording and editing, can simply input a script and let ElevenLabs produce a perfect audio clone of their voice. This technology not only saves time but also allows the podcaster to experiment with different styles and voices, making their content more engaging and diverse.

Suno: Consider a music enthusiast who dreams of creating their own songs but lacks the technical skills to do so. With Suno, they can simply type in a prompt like "create a Justin Bieber-style pop song about AI in the workplace," and within seconds, they have a fully produced track. This level of accessibility could lead to a surge in amateur musicians and a diverse array of new music.

Speechify: Think about a student with dyslexia who struggles to read lengthy textbooks. Speechify can convert these texts into audio, allowing the student to listen and learn more effectively.

This tool not only enhances accessibility but also empowers individuals with disabilities to access information more easily.

Chapter 7: Autonomous AI Agents

Current State

Autonomous AI agents capable of performing complex tasks are becoming more prevalent. These agents go beyond simple interactions, performing functions such as making reservations, planning trips, and connecting to other services. The rise of autonomous AI signifies a shift towards more intelligent and capable systems, enhancing efficiency and convenience in various applications.

Future Expectations

The future will see even more advanced autonomous AI agents with greater capabilities and autonomy. These agents will be able to handle more complex and diverse tasks, learning and adapting to new situations with minimal human intervention. Advances in natural language processing and machine learning will enable more seamless and intuitive interactions between humans and AI agents.

Positive Implications

1. *Increased Convenience:* Autonomous AI agents can handle routine tasks, making daily life more convenient and freeing up time for more important activities.

2. *Enhanced Efficiency:* By automating complex tasks, autonomous AI agents can increase efficiency in various applications, from customer service to logistics.

3. *Personalised Experiences:* Autonomous AI agents can provide personalised services tailored to individual preferences and needs.

Negative Implications

1. *Privacy Concerns:* The use of autonomous AI agents raises concerns about data privacy and the potential misuse of personal information.

2. *Job Displacement:* As autonomous AI agents take over more tasks, there is a risk that certain jobs may become obsolete, leading to economic and social challenges.

3. *Dependency Risks:* Over-reliance on autonomous AI agents can lead to a loss of essential skills and reduce human agency in decision-making.

Examples

Personal Assistants: AI-powered personal assistants like Google Assistant, Amazon Alexa, and Apple Siri are becoming increasingly capable of managing daily tasks. These assistants can schedule appointments, set reminders, and even control smart home devices, making life more convenient for users.

Customer Service Bots: Many companies are using AI chatbots to handle customer service inquiries. These bots can provide quick and accurate responses to common questions, freeing up human agents to handle more complex issues. This not only improves efficiency but also enhances the customer experience.

Autonomous Vehicles: Self-driving cars, like those being developed by Tesla and Waymo, are an example of autonomous AI agents in transportation. These vehicles can navigate roads, avoid obstacles, and make decisions in real-time, potentially reducing traffic accidents and improving transportation efficiency.

Chapter 8: AI in Robotics

Current State

As was discussed in Chapter 5, the integration of AI with robotics has led to significant advancements in robotic capabilities. AI-powered robots are becoming more flexible, capable, and interactive, transforming various industries and applications. Language models like PaLM-E and RT-2 enhance robotic capabilities, enabling natural language understanding and autonomous operation. These advancements open up new possibilities for automation in industries ranging from manufacturing to healthcare.

Future Expectations

Future developments in AI robotics will likely focus on increasing the autonomy and intelligence of robots. This includes improvements in robot dexterity, adaptability, and decision-making capabilities. Collaborative robots (cobots) that can work alongside humans in various settings will become more prevalent. Additionally, advancements in human-robot interaction will lead to more intuitive and seamless collaboration between humans and robots.

Positive Implications

1. *Increased Efficiency:* AI-powered robots can perform tasks more efficiently and accurately than humans, leading to increased productivity in various industries.

2. *Enhanced Safety:* Robots can take on dangerous tasks, reducing the risk of injury to human workers.

3. *Improved Quality of Life:* In healthcare, AI-powered robots can assist with surgeries, rehabilitation, and elderly care, improving patient outcomes and quality of life.

Negative Implications

1. *Job Displacement:* The widespread adoption of AI-powered robots may lead to job losses, particularly in industries that rely heavily on manual labour.

2. *Ethical Concerns:* The use of robots in sensitive areas such as healthcare and caregiving raises ethical concerns about human dignity and the quality of care.

3. *Security Risks:* Autonomous robots are vulnerable to hacking and other security threats, which could have serious consequences in critical applications. There are also the concerns of malevolent AI – this topic is discussed further in chapter 19.

Examples

Factory Automation: In manufacturing, AI-powered robots are revolutionising production lines. Companies like Tesla use advanced robotics for assembling cars, improving precision and speed while reducing labour costs. These robots can work around the clock without fatigue, significantly boosting productivity.

Healthcare Robotics: In healthcare, robots like the da Vinci Surgical System are assisting surgeons in performing complex procedures with greater precision. These robots provide enhanced visualisation and control, leading to better patient outcomes and shorter recovery times. Additionally, robots like TUG can autonomously transport medical supplies within hospitals, reducing the workload on healthcare staff.

Service Robots: In the service industry, robots like SoftBank's Pepper are being used to interact with customers, provide information, and even offer companionship. These robots can recognise faces, understand speech, and respond to queries, making them valuable assets in retail, hospitality, and healthcare settings.

Chapter 9: AI in the Workplace

Current State

It is not just robots that are enhancing productivity in the workplace, other aspects of AI are also enhancing efficiency and effectiveness in various tasks. Platforms like GitHub Copilot, Taskade, and Motion exemplify how AI can improve coding, task management, and scheduling. GitHub Copilot offers intelligent code suggestions and error fixes, while Taskade and Motion provide AI-powered project planning and task rescheduling. These tools streamline workflows, allowing users to focus on strategic activities and boosting overall productivity.

Future Expectations

Future AI productivity tools will become even more integrated into daily workflows, offering more advanced features and greater customisation. AI will be able to anticipate users' needs and provide proactive assistance, further enhancing productivity. Collaborative AI tools that facilitate teamwork and communication will become more prevalent, transforming how people work together.

The future of the workplace is discussed further in section 4 of this book.

Positive Implications

1. *Enhanced Efficiency:* AI-powered productivity tools can automate routine tasks, freeing up time for more strategic and creative work.

2. *Improved Collaboration:* AI tools can facilitate better communication and collaboration among team members, leading to more effective teamwork.

3. *Increased Innovation:* By reducing the time spent on mundane tasks, AI productivity tools can spur innovation and creativity.

Negative Implications

1. *Dependence on Technology:* Over-reliance on AI tools can lead to a loss of essential skills and reduce human agency in decision-making.

2. *Privacy Concerns:* The use of AI productivity tools raises concerns about data privacy and the potential misuse of personal information.

3. *Job Displacement:* As AI takes over more tasks, there is a risk that certain jobs may become obsolete, leading to economic and social challenges.

Examples

GitHub Copilot: This tool assists software developers by providing real-time code suggestions and error fixes. By automating routine coding tasks, GitHub Copilot allows developers to focus on more complex aspects of software development, speeding up the development process and improving code quality.

Taskade: An AI-powered project management tool that helps teams plan, organise, and execute projects more efficiently. It offers features like automated task scheduling, real-time collaboration, and intelligent reminders, making project management more streamlined and effective.

Motion: Motion is an AI-powered productivity tool that helps users manage their schedules and tasks. By analysing users' habits and priorities, Motion can automatically reschedule tasks and meetings, ensuring that important tasks are prioritised, and deadlines are met.

Chapter 10: Regulation and Policy

Current State

Significant strides have been made in AI regulation and policy, particularly in the European Union and the United States. The EU is leading with comprehensive AI regulations focusing on transparency, accountability, and consumer protection. In the U.S., executive actions and legislative efforts, such as the CREATE AI Act, aim to broaden access to AI resources and promote responsible development. These regulatory frameworks are essential for guiding the ethical and safe deployment of AI technologies.

Future Expectations

Future AI regulations will likely become more comprehensive and globally harmonised, moving towards consistent standards and practices across different regions. International cooperation on AI policy will become increasingly important, as the global nature of AI development necessitates coordinated efforts. New regulations will likely seek to address emerging issues such as AI in military applications, autonomous weapons, and AI's role in surveillance and privacy.

Positive Implications

1. *Consumer Protection:* Strong regulations can protect consumers from potential harms associated with AI, such as privacy violations and biased decision-making.

2. *Ethical Development:* Regulatory frameworks can ensure that AI technologies are developed and deployed ethically, minimising risks and maximising benefits.

3. *Global Standards:* Harmonised global standards can facilitate international collaboration and innovation in AI.

Negative Implications

1. *Regulatory Burden:* Compliance with complex regulations can be burdensome for companies, particularly small and medium-sized enterprises.

2. *Innovation Stifling:* Overly stringent regulations may stifle innovation and slow down the development of new AI technologies.

3. *Geopolitical Tensions:* Differing regulatory approaches between regions can lead to geopolitical tensions and conflicts over AI governance.

Examples

The EU AI Act: The European Union is at the forefront of AI regulation with its proposed AI Act. This legislation aims to create a regulatory framework for AI, focusing on high-risk applications and ensuring that AI systems are safe, transparent, and accountable. The AI Act sets out stringent requirements for

AI developers, including rigorous testing, documentation, and oversight.

The CREATE AI Act: In the United States, the CREATE AI Act is a legislative effort to broaden access to AI resources and promote responsible AI development. This act aims to provide funding for AI research and development, support AI education and workforce training, and establish ethical guidelines for AI use.

Global AI Governance: The Organisation for Economic Co-operation and Development (OECD) has established principles for AI governance that emphasise transparency, accountability, and human-centred values. These principles provide a foundation for international cooperation on AI regulation, ensuring that AI technologies are developed and used in ways that benefit society as a whole.

Chapter 11: Responsible AI

Current State

The responsible development and deployment of AI systems has become a critical focal point in recent years. Issues such as data privacy, algorithmic bias, transparency, and security are at the forefront of discussions about AI ethics. Companies are increasingly required to ensure that their AI systems comply with data protection regulations and maintain transparency about how data is collected, used, and stored. Researchers and developers are focusing on creating more inclusive datasets and developing algorithms that can detect and mitigate bias.

Future Expectations

In the future, responsible AI practices will likely become more standardised, with stricter regulations and guidelines to ensure ethical AI development. Advances in explainable AI will make it easier for users to understand how AI systems make decisions, increasing transparency and accountability. Additionally, new frameworks for ethical AI design will be developed, ensuring that AI systems are not only effective but also fair and just.

Positive Implications

1. *Increased Trust*: By prioritising transparency and fairness, responsible AI practices can help build public trust in AI technologies.

2. *Fairer Systems*: Efforts to address bias and ensure fairness in AI systems can lead to more equitable outcomes, particularly in critical areas such as hiring and lending.

3. *Improved Security*: Enhancing the security of AI systems can prevent misuse and protect against adversarial attacks, ensuring the safety and reliability of AI technologies.

Negative Implications

1. *Compliance Costs:* Implementing responsible AI practices can be costly and time-consuming, particularly for smaller companies or startups.

2. *Ethical Dilemmas:* Balancing the need for transparency with privacy concerns can be challenging, and ethical dilemmas may arise when making decisions about AI design and deployment.

3. *Potential for Misuse:* Despite best efforts, there is always a risk that AI systems could be misused or manipulated, leading to harmful outcomes.

Examples

Data Privacy Regulations: In Europe, the General Data Protection Regulation (GDPR) sets strict guidelines on how companies must handle personal data. This regulation has pushed AI developers to prioritise data privacy and transparency, ensuring that users are informed about how their data is used and have control over it.

Algorithmic Fairness: Companies like Google and IBM are actively working on algorithms that detect and mitigate bias. For example, IBM's AI Fairness 360 toolkit provides developers with resources to assess and improve the fairness of their AI models, ensuring that decisions made by AI are equitable.

AI Transparency: Explainable AI (XAI) is a growing field focused on making AI decisions more understandable to humans. This involves developing models that provide clear and interpretable explanations for their decisions, helping users trust and validate the outputs of AI systems.

Chapter 12: AI Misuse and Incidents

Current State

Tracking and addressing the misuse of AI technologies is crucial. The AI Incident Database (which catalogues incidents where artificial intelligence (AI) systems have caused harm or exhibited undesirable behaviour) highlights the increasing number of incidents related to AI misuse, emphasising the need for robust safety and security measures.

The race between detection and avoidance in AI misuse is an ongoing and dynamic struggle that highlights the dual nature of technological advancements. On one side, detection involves developing sophisticated AI systems capable of identifying malicious activities, such as deepfakes (see next chapter), cyberattacks, and fraudulent behaviours. These detection systems leverage advanced machine learning techniques, anomaly detection algorithms, and vast datasets to recognise and counteract harmful actions effectively.

However, as detection capabilities improve, bad actors continually evolve their methods to evade these systems, employing increasingly sophisticated techniques to bypass security measures and mask their activities. This cat-and-mouse game drives a continuous cycle of innovation, where each advancement in detection prompts a corresponding advancement in avoidance tactics.

The stakes are high, as the balance between detection and avoidance impacts not only cybersecurity but also trust in AI applications across various domains, from finance and healthcare to national security and personal privacy. As such, ongoing research, collaboration, and investment in AI ethics and security are crucial to staying ahead in this race, ensuring that the benefits of AI are not overshadowed by its potential for misuse.

Future Expectations

Future efforts to address AI misuse will focus on developing more robust safety and security frameworks, increasing transparency, and enhancing accountability. Advances in AI detection technologies will help identify and mitigate misuse, while regulatory efforts will seek to ensure that AI technologies are used ethically and responsibly. Collaboration between tech companies, governments, and researchers will be essential in addressing the risks associated with AI misuse.

Positive Implications

1. *Improved Safety:* Enhanced safety and security measures can prevent AI misuse and protect against harmful outcomes.

2. *Increased Accountability:* Greater transparency and accountability in AI development and deployment can build public trust and ensure ethical practices.

3. *Proactive Mitigation:* Ongoing vigilance and proactive measures can identify and mitigate risks before they result in serious incidents.

Negative Implications

1. *Regulatory Challenges*: Developing effective regulations to address AI misuse can be challenging, particularly in a rapidly evolving field.

2. *Resource Constraints:* Implementing robust safety and security measures can be costly and resource-intensive, particularly for smaller companies or startups.

3. *Unintended* Consequences: Efforts to address AI misuse may have unintended consequences, such as stifling innovation or creating new ethical dilemmas.

Examples

Bias in Hiring Algorithms: There have been instances where AI algorithms used in hiring processes have demonstrated bias against certain groups. For example, an AI system used by a major tech company was found to favor male candidates over female candidates. Addressing such biases is critical for ensuring fair and equitable outcomes.

Autonomous Weapon Systems: The use of AI in military applications, such as autonomous weapon systems, raises significant ethical and security concerns. These systems can make life-and-death decisions without human intervention, leading to debates about the moral implications of their use.

AI-Driven Surveillance: The use of AI for surveillance purposes can lead to privacy violations and civil liberties concerns. For example, facial recognition technology has been used by law enforcement agencies to monitor public spaces, raising questions about the balance between security and privacy.

Conclusion

The future of AI holds immense potential to transform human society across various domains. As AI technologies continue to advance, they will drive economic growth, revolutionise healthcare, and enhance daily life, while also posing significant ethical and social challenges. Preparing for this future requires a balanced approach that fosters innovation while addressing the potential risks and implications of AI.

Chapter 13: Deepfakes

Current State

Deepfake technology has become a major concern, with AI-generated videos and audio posing significant challenges for authenticity and trust. Deepfakes can make individuals appear to say or do things they haven't, raising concerns about disinformation and personal reputations.

The rise of deepfake technology has not only enabled the creation of realistic yet fabricated content but has also given bad actors a new defence mechanism - the ability to dismiss genuine recordings as deepfakes. By casting doubt on authentic evidence, individuals facing incrimination - such as politicians, business leaders, or criminals - can claim that a legitimate video or audio recording is, in fact, a manipulated deepfake. This tactic undermines trust in real evidence, complicating efforts to hold individuals accountable, and eroding the public's confidence in digital media as a reliable source of truth. As the lines between real and fake blur, the deepfake defence becomes a powerful tool for evasion, turning the technology's original threat on its head.

Efforts to detect and mitigate deepfakes are ongoing, involving advanced machine learning techniques to identify manipulated content.

Future Expectations

The future will likely see more sophisticated and harder-to-detect deepfakes, necessitating continuous advancements in detection technologies. Regulatory efforts will increase to address the malicious use of deepfakes, and public awareness campaigns will educate people about the risks and how to identify fake content. Collaboration between tech companies, governments, and researchers will be crucial in combating the spread of deepfakes.

Positive Implications

1. *Innovative Applications:* Deepfake technology can be used for positive purposes, such as in the entertainment industry for creating realistic special effects or in education for immersive learning experiences.

2. *Enhanced Detection:* Continuous improvements in detection technologies can help mitigate the risks associated with deepfakes.

Negative Implications

1. *Disinformation:* Deepfakes can be used to spread false information and manipulate public opinion, undermining trust in media and institutions.

2. *Privacy Violations:* The creation of deepfake content without individuals' consent can violate their privacy and harm their reputations.

3. *Security Threats*: Deepfakes can be used in cyberattacks, fraud, and other malicious activities, posing significant security risks.

Examples

Political Deepfakes: During election campaigns, deepfakes can be used to create fake videos of candidates making controversial statements. These videos can quickly go viral, spreading disinformation and influencing voter opinions. Detecting and debunking these deepfakes is crucial for maintaining the integrity of democratic processes.

Celebrity Deepfakes: Celebrities are often targeted by deepfakes, with fake videos being created for malicious purposes such as blackmail or defamation. For example, a deepfake video of a celebrity saying or doing something scandalous can damage their reputation and career. Efforts to protect celebrities from such malicious attacks are essential.

Educational Uses: On a positive note, deepfake technology can be used in education to create realistic simulations for training purposes. For instance, medical students can use deepfake simulations to practice surgical procedures in a controlled environment, enhancing their skills and preparedness.

Chapter 14: AI and Elections

Current State

AI's influence on political processes and elections is a growing concern. AI is used in political campaigns to analyse voter data, craft targeted messages, and optimise campaign strategies. This allows political campaigns to reach voters more effectively but also raises concerns about privacy and the potential for manipulation. The use of AI-generated disinformation, such as deepfake videos, poses significant risks to election integrity.

Future Expectations

Future elections will see even more sophisticated use of AI in campaign strategies, voter analysis, and targeted messaging. Regulatory efforts will increase to ensure the ethical use of AI in elections and to prevent manipulation and disinformation. Advances in AI detection technologies will help identify and mitigate the impact of AI-generated disinformation.

Positive Implications

1. *Informed Campaigns:* AI can help political campaigns understand voter preferences and concerns, leading to more informed and relevant campaign strategies.

2. *Efficient Resource Allocation:* AI can optimise campaign resource allocation, ensuring that efforts are focused where they are most needed.

Negative Implications

1. *Privacy Violations:* The use of AI to analyse voter data raises significant privacy concerns and the potential for misuse of personal information.

2. *Manipulation and Disinformation:* AI-generated disinformation can undermine the integrity of elections and manipulate public opinion, posing a threat to democracy.

3. *Inequality in Campaigning:* The use of advanced AI technologies in campaigns can create inequalities, giving well-funded campaigns an unfair advantage – although it could be argued that this is nothing new!

Examples

Cambridge Analytica Scandal: In the 2016 U.S. presidential election, Cambridge Analytica used AI to analyse and exploit voter data, creating highly targeted and manipulative campaign ads. This scandal highlighted the potential for AI to be used unethically in elections, leading to widespread calls for better regulation and oversight.

Deepfake Campaign Ads: In recent elections, there have been instances of deepfake videos being used to spread disinformation about candidates. These videos can be highly convincing, making it difficult for voters to discern fact from fiction. Detecting and countering such deepfakes is crucial for maintaining election integrity.

AI-Driven Voter Outreach: On a positive note, AI can be used to enhance voter outreach efforts. For example, AI chatbots can engage with voters, answer their questions, and provide information about voting procedures. This can help increase voter participation and ensure that more people have access to accurate information.

Chapter 15: Hardware and Infrastructure

Current State

The development and deployment of AI technologies depends heavily on hardware infrastructure. With a global shortage of GPU processors posing significant challenges and energy demands pressurising power supply, companies (and countries) are competing for these resources, driving efforts to develop low-power alternatives and increase production capacity. Innovations in AI hardware is essential to democratise access to AI capabilities and sustain the pace of AI advancements.

Future Expectations

Future developments in AI hardware will focus on increasing efficiency, reducing costs, and improving accessibility. Advances in quantum computing, neuromorphic computing, and other innovative technologies will provide new opportunities for AI development. Efforts to address the GPU shortage may well lead to the development of alternative hardware solutions that can support AI application.

Positive Implications

1. *Enhanced Performance:* Advances in AI hardware will lead to more powerful and efficient AI systems, enabling new applications and capabilities.

2. *Increased Accessibility:* Innovative hardware solutions can democratise access to AI technologies, making them available to a broader range of users.

3. *Sustainable Development:* Developing low-power and energy-efficient AI hardware can reduce the environmental impact of AI technologies.

Negative Implications

1. *Resource Competition:* The competition for AI hardware resources can create inequalities and hinder the development of AI technologies in less affluent regions.

2. *Security Risks:* Advances in AI hardware can also pose security risks, as more powerful AI systems can be used for malicious purposes. These security risks are expanded on further in some of the scenarios shown in section 5.

3. *Environmental* Impact: The production and disposal of AI hardware can have significant environmental consequences, necessitating sustainable practices.

Examples

NVIDIA GPUs: NVIDIA is a leading manufacturer of GPUs, which are essential for running AI applications. However, the global shortage of these processors has led to increased prices and limited availability, impacting the development and deployment of AI technologies. Efforts to increase production and develop alternative hardware solutions are crucial for sustaining AI advancements.

Quantum Computing: Companies like IBM and Google are making significant strides in quantum computing, which promises to revolutionise AI by providing exponentially greater processing power. Quantum computers can solve complex problems that are currently too complex, opening up new possibilities for AI research and applications.

Neuromorphic Computing: Neuromorphic computing is an emerging field that aims to mimic the human brain's neural architecture to create more efficient and powerful AI systems. Companies like Intel are developing neuromorphic chips that can perform AI tasks with lower power consumption and greater efficiency, paving the way for more sustainable AI technologies.

Our AI Journey

SECTION 4 – THE FUTURE OF AI AND HUMAN SOCIETY

This section delves into the transformative potential of artificial intelligence and its impact on the most pressing challenges facing human society. From addressing wealth disparity and climate change, to mitigating the impacts of war and guiding ethical development, this section explores how AI technologies could reshape our world.

The chapters address the complex relationship between AI and governance, highlighting the critical role of governments in ensuring that AI is deployed ethically and inclusively. This includes an exploration of the risks associated with malevolent AI, especially when integrated into robotics, and the challenges AI development faces due to energy, material, and computational constraints.

By providing a comprehensive view of AI's potential, challenges, and solutions, this section aims to offer a roadmap for leveraging AI responsibly to create a more equitable, sustainable, and secure future.

Chapter 16: The Potential for AI to Address Key Challenges in Human Society

Artificial intelligence (AI) holds immense potential to tackle some of the most pressing challenges facing human society today. From addressing wealth disparity and climate change to mitigating the impacts of war, AI technologies could play a transformative role in creating a more equitable, sustainable, and peaceful world. This section explores how AI might contribute to these critical areas, offering innovative solutions and driving positive change.

Addressing Wealth Disparity

Wealth disparity, both within countries and between them, is a significant issue that exacerbates social and economic inequalities. AI has the potential to bridge these gaps by promoting financial inclusion, improving access to education, and supporting the implementation of policies like universal basic income (UBI).

Financial Inclusion and Access to Services

AI-powered financial technologies (fintech) can provide unbanked and underbanked populations with access to financial services. For example, mobile banking apps powered by AI can offer microloans, credit scoring, and personalised financial advice to individuals who lack traditional banking services. Companies like Tala and Branch use AI to assess creditworthiness and provide loans to people in developing countries, enabling them to invest in their businesses and improve their livelihoods.

Personalised Education and Skill Development

AI can democratise access to quality education by providing personalised learning experiences tailored to individual needs. AI-driven platforms like Coursera and Khan Academy use machine learning algorithms to recommend courses, track progress, and offer personalised feedback, helping learners acquire new skills and improve their employability. By making education more accessible and effective, AI can help reduce wealth disparities by empowering individuals to achieve their economic potential.

Universal Basic Income (UBI) Implementation

AI can support the implementation and management of UBI programmes by ensuring efficient and equitable distribution of funds. AI systems can analyse economic data to determine optimal UBI amounts and identify eligible recipients. Additionally, AI can help monitor and prevent fraud, ensuring that resources are directed to those who need them most. Pilot programmes in countries like Finland and Kenya have demonstrated the potential benefits of UBI in reducing poverty and promoting economic stability.

Combatting Climate Change

Climate change is one of the most urgent challenges facing humanity. AI can play a critical role in mitigating the impacts of climate change by optimising energy use, enhancing environmental monitoring and carbon capture technology, and supporting the transition to renewable energy sources.

Optimising Energy Consumption

AI can improve energy efficiency in various sectors, from industrial processes to household energy use. Smart grids, powered by AI, can optimise electricity distribution by predicting demand and adjusting supply in real-time. AI-driven systems like Google's DeepMind have successfully reduced the energy consumption of data centres by optimising cooling processes, demonstrating significant potential for energy savings in other applications.

AI algorithms are also being used by logistics providers to analyse vast amounts of data to determine the most efficient routes for delivery vehicles. This includes real-time traffic data, historical traffic patterns, weather conditions, and delivery time windows. By continuously learning from this data, AI can dynamically adjust routes to avoid delays and reduce fuel consumption. For example, UPS uses an AI-based system called ORION (On-Road Integrated Optimization and Navigation) which processes data from more than 250 million address points. ORION has helped UPS save millions of miles driven annually, and reduced fuel consumption (and cost) significantly.

Enhancing Environmental Monitoring

AI-powered remote sensing and data analysis can provide valuable insights into environmental changes. AI algorithms can analyse satellite imagery, sensor data, and climate models to monitor deforestation, track wildlife populations, and predict natural disasters. These insights can inform conservation efforts and policy decisions, helping to protect ecosystems and biodiversity. Projects like Global Forest Watch use AI to monitor forests in real-time, enabling rapid response to illegal logging and other environmental threats.

Supporting Renewable Energy Transition

AI can accelerate the adoption of renewable energy sources by optimising their integration into the power grid. AI algorithms can predict weather patterns to improve the reliability of solar and wind energy, balance supply and demand, and manage energy storage systems.

Enhancement of Carbon Capture Technology

Artificial intelligence is also increasingly being employed to enhance the efficiency and effectiveness of carbon capture technologies including: -

> *Optimisation of Carbon Capture Processes* - AI is used to optimise the parameters and operations of carbon capture systems, ensuring they operate at maximum efficiency. By analysing vast amounts of data from sensors and process controls, AI algorithms can identify the optimal conditions for capturing CO_2 from industrial emissions. This includes adjusting variables like temperature, pressure, and flow rates in real-time. Researchers at the University of Toronto have developed an AI-driven approach to optimise the design and operation of CO_2 capture materials, leading to significant improvements in their performance.

> *Machine Learning for Material Discovery* - Machine learning algorithms are used to discover and design new materials for carbon capture. These materials, such as metal-organic frameworks (MOFs) and advanced solvents, are critical for efficiently capturing CO_2 from various sources. AI can rapidly screen and predict the performance of thousands of potential materials, significantly speeding up the discovery process. MIT researchers have employed machine learning to identify MOFs that can capture CO_2 more effectively than traditional materials, reducing the time required to discover new materials from years to months.

> *Predictive Maintenance* - AI-driven predictive maintenance helps ensure that carbon capture facilities operate without

unexpected downtimes. By analysing data from equipment sensors, AI can predict when maintenance is needed before a failure occurs, thereby reducing operational costs and increasing the reliability of carbon capture systems. Siemens has developed AI-based predictive maintenance solutions for carbon capture facilities, which use machine learning algorithms to monitor equipment health and predict failures.

Data Analytics and Simulation - AI is used to analyse complex data sets from carbon capture processes and simulate different scenarios to improve efficiency and effectiveness. This includes modelling the behaviour of CO_2 under different conditions and predicting the impact of various operational changes on capture rates and energy consumption. The National Energy Technology Laboratory (NETL) in the United States uses AI and advanced data analytics to model and simulate carbon capture processes, aiming to identify the most efficient and cost-effective methods for large-scale implementation.

Integration with Renewable Energy - AI helps integrate carbon capture technologies with renewable energy sources, optimising the use of fluctuating power supplies from wind and solar to power carbon capture systems. This integration is crucial for reducing the carbon footprint of the capture process itself. Researchers are developing AI algorithms that manage the power supply for carbon capture facilities by predicting renewable energy availability and adjusting operations accordingly, ensuring efficient use of renewable energy while maximising CO_2 capture.

Real-Time Monitoring and Control - AI technologies enable real-time monitoring and control of carbon capture processes. This includes using AI to continuously analyse data from sensors and make real-time adjustments to maintain optimal performance. Carbon Clean Solutions, a company specialising in carbon capture technologies, uses AI for real-time monitoring and control of their systems, improving capture efficiency and reducing operational costs.

Conclusion

Artificial Intelligence offers transformative solutions for some of the most critical challenges facing society today, including wealth disparity and climate change.

By leveraging AI technologies, we can promote financial inclusion, enhance education, and support policies like universal basic income (UBI) to empower underserved populations. AI-powered fintech, personalised education platforms, and UBI management systems demonstrate how technology can be harnessed to create economic stability and opportunity, helping to close the gap between different socio-economic groups.

AI will play a crucial role in environmental sustainability, optimising energy consumption, enhancing environmental monitoring, and supporting the transition to renewable energy. The advancements in carbon capture technology showcase how AI can optimise processes, discover new materials, and integrate with renewable energy sources to mitigate climate change effectively. The chapter highlights how, when used responsibly and innovatively, AI has the potential to create a more equitable, sustainable, and resilient future for human society.

Chapter 17: AI's Impact on Society: The Hollywood Strikes

The recent Hollywood strikes by writers and actors have brought to the forefront the profound impact of artificial intelligence (AI) on the entertainment industry and society at large. These strikes highlight the growing concerns and debates surrounding the integration of AI in creative fields and its implications for jobs, creativity, and the future of work.

Background of the Strikes

In 2023, Hollywood witnessed significant labour actions as members of the Writers Guild of America (WGA) and the Screen Actors Guild-American Federation of Television and Radio Artists (SAG-AFTRA) went on strike. One of the core issues driving these strikes was the use of AI in the entertainment industry. Writers and actors expressed deep concerns about how AI technologies could replace human creativity and labour, potentially leading to job losses and changes in how creative work is valued and produced.

Key Concerns

Job Displacement: Writers and actors fear that AI could be used to generate scripts, dialogues, and even digital representations of actors, effectively reducing the need for human talent. This could lead to widespread job losses and undermine the livelihoods of thousands of professionals in the industry.

Creative Integrity: There is a concern that AI-generated content may lack the depth, nuance, and originality that human writers and actors bring to their work. The fear is that reliance on AI could lead to a homogenisation of content, with formulaic and less innovative outputs dominating the industry.

Ethical Use of AI: The ethical implications of using AI in creative processes are significant. Writers and actors are advocating for clear guidelines and regulations to ensure that AI is used responsibly and that the contributions of human creators are recognised and fairly compensated.

Examples

Netflix's AI Job Listing: A job listing by Netflix for an AI specialist with a high salary sparked outrage among Hollywood unions, highlighting the fears of AI replacing human jobs. This incident underscored the need for transparency and dialogue about AI's role in the industry.

Digital Avatars and Deepfakes: The use of digital avatars and deepfake technology has raised questions about authenticity and consent. Actors are particularly concerned about the potential misuse of their likenesses without adequate compensation or control.

Industry Response

The entertainment industry has been grappling with these issues, and the strikes have prompted discussions about how to balance the benefits of AI with the need to protect human jobs and creativity. Some key developments include:

Collective Bargaining Agreements: The recent agreements between studios and unions have included provisions addressing the use of AI. These agreements aim to ensure that AI is used in ways that complement rather than replace human labour, and that there are safeguards to protect jobs and creative rights.

Ethical AI Initiatives: Industry stakeholders are increasingly calling for ethical guidelines and standards for AI use. Organisations like the World Economic Forum have been involved in discussions about human-centred AI, emphasising the need for responsible AI integration in creative industries.

Investment in Human-AI Collaboration: Rather than seeing AI as a threat, there is a growing emphasis on exploring how AI can enhance human creativity and productivity. This includes using AI to handle repetitive tasks, allowing writers and actors to focus on more complex and creative aspects of their work.

Conclusion

The entertainment sector's experience underscores the need for proactive regulation, ethical considerations, and a balanced approach to integrating technological innovation with human-centred values. The Hollywood strikes are part of a broader conversation about AI's impact on society, as the rapid advancement of AI is likely to raise similar issues in other industries. By advocating for ethical AI practices, fair compensation, and the protection of jobs, writers and actors have set a precedent for other sectors navigating the complex interplay between AI and human labour. The outcome of these strikes and the ongoing dialogue will be crucial in shaping the future of work in an AI-driven world.

Our AI Journey

Chapter 18: Mitigating the Impacts of War

War and conflict have devastating effects on human lives and societies. AI can contribute to peacebuilding and conflict resolution by providing early warning systems, enhancing humanitarian efforts, and supporting post-conflict reconstruction.

Early Warning Systems for Conflict Prevention

AI can analyse social media, news reports, and other data sources to identify patterns and indicators of potential conflicts. By providing early warnings, AI systems can help governments and international organisations take proactive measures to prevent violence. For example, the United Nations has explored the use of AI to detect early signs of political instability and social unrest, enabling timely intervention.

Enhancing Humanitarian Aid

In conflict zones, AI can enhance the effectiveness of humanitarian aid by improving logistics, resource allocation, and communication. AI-powered drones and robotics can deliver supplies to remote or dangerous areas, while machine learning algorithms can optimise the distribution of resources based on real-time data. Organisations like the World Food Programme use AI to forecast food shortages and coordinate relief efforts, ensuring that aid reaches those in need.

Supporting Post-Conflict Reconstruction

AI can assist in post-conflict reconstruction by facilitating infrastructure rebuilding, economic recovery, and social reconciliation. AI-driven tools can help map and clear landmines, reconstruct damaged buildings using 3D printing, and provide mental health support through AI-powered chatbots and virtual therapy. By leveraging AI, post-conflict societies can rebuild more effectively and sustainably, fostering long-term peace and stability.

Conclusion

AI holds significant potential to mitigate the devastating impacts of war by providing innovative solutions for conflict prevention, humanitarian aid, and post-conflict reconstruction. Through early warning systems that analyse social media and news data, AI can help identify signs of political instability, enabling governments and international organisations to take proactive measures to prevent violence. Additionally, AI-powered tools enhance the effectiveness of humanitarian aid by optimising resource distribution and facilitating the delivery of supplies in dangerous areas. In post-conflict environments, AI assists with clearing landmines, rebuilding infrastructure, and supporting mental health through AI-driven therapy solutions, ultimately contributing to long-term peace and stability.

As AI continues to advance, it is essential to ensure that its deployment in conflict scenarios is ethical, inclusive, and geared toward fostering peace and recovery in war-torn regions.

Chapter 19: Risk of Malevolent AI Including Incorporation in Robotics

The potential for malevolent AI, particularly when integrated into robotics, poses significant risks to society. These risks can arise from intentional misuse by malicious actors or unintentional consequences due to flawed design, implementation, or insufficient oversight. Here's an overview of the key risks associated with malevolent AI in robotics:

Autonomous Weapons

Scenario: AI-controlled robots and drones are used as autonomous weapons by military forces or rogue actors.

Impact: Autonomous weapons could make decisions to harm humans without human intervention, leading to ethical dilemmas and potentially large-scale loss of life. The proliferation of such weapons could also spark an arms race, increasing global instability.

Cybersecurity Threats

Scenario: AI-powered robots are hacked or manipulated by cybercriminals.

Impact: Hackers could take control of AI robots, causing them to perform harmful actions or access sensitive information. This could lead to physical harm, property damage, and breaches of privacy.

Surveillance and Privacy Violations

Scenario: AI robots are used for mass surveillance by authoritarian regimes or corporations.

Impact: The use of AI in surveillance can lead to severe privacy violations and the suppression of civil liberties. Constant monitoring by AI robots can create an environment of fear and control, stifling freedom of expression and movement.

Bias and Discrimination

Scenario: AI algorithms embedded in robots exhibit biased behaviour due to flawed training data.

Impact: Biased AI systems can lead to discriminatory actions by robots, such as unfair treatment in law enforcement, healthcare, or customer service. This can perpetuate social inequalities and erode trust in AI technologies.

Unintended Consequences

Scenario: AI robots make decisions that result in unintended harm due to flawed programming or insufficient understanding of complex environments.

Impact: Robots operating in critical areas like healthcare, transportation, and industrial settings could cause accidents or failures, leading to injuries, loss of life, or significant economic damage.

Loss of Control

Scenario: Highly autonomous AI systems in robots act unpredictably or beyond human control.

Impact: If robots become too autonomous, they might perform actions that are not aligned with human intentions or values, leading to dangerous situations. Ensuring that humans can always override AI decisions is crucial to maintaining control.

Weaponisation by Non-State Actors

Scenario: Terrorist groups or criminal organisations use AI robots for malicious purposes.

Impact: AI robots could be weaponised to conduct attacks, disrupt infrastructure, or create chaos. The accessibility of AI technology increases the risk of its use by non-state actors with malicious intent.

Mitigation Strategies

Robust Security Measures: Implementing strong cybersecurity protocols to protect AI systems and robots from hacking and unauthorised access.

Ethical Design Principles: Incorporating ethical guidelines in the design and deployment of AI robots to prevent biases and ensure fairness.

Human Oversight and Control: Ensuring that AI robots are designed with mechanisms for human intervention and control to prevent unintended actions.

Regulatory Frameworks: Developing and enforcing regulations that govern the use of AI in robotics, particularly in sensitive areas like autonomous weapons and surveillance.

Transparency and Accountability: Promoting transparency in AI algorithms and holding developers and operators accountable for the actions of AI robots.

International Cooperation: Encouraging international collaboration to address the global risks posed by malevolent AI and ensure the responsible development and use of AI technologies.

Conclusion

The risks associated with malevolent AI in robotics are substantial and multifaceted, encompassing cybersecurity threats, ethical dilemmas, and the potential for large-scale harm. Addressing these risks requires a concerted effort from developers, policymakers, and international organisations to implement robust safeguards, ethical guidelines, and regulatory frameworks. By proactively managing these risks, we can harness the benefits of AI in robotics while minimising the potential for misuse and unintended consequences.

Chapter 20: AI and Governments: Supporting the Achievement of Societal Challenges

Governments play a crucial role in harnessing the power of AI to address significant societal challenges, including wealth disparity, climate change, and conflict. By creating conducive policies, investing in AI research and development, and promoting ethical and inclusive AI use, governments might seek to ensure that AI technologies are deployed effectively for the greater good. This section explores how governments could support and accelerate the achievement of these critical goals.

Policy and Regulation

Governments can establish comprehensive policies and regulations that encourage the responsible development and deployment of AI technologies. These policies should address ethical concerns, ensure data privacy, and promote global alignment, fairness and transparency in AI systems.

Ethical AI Frameworks

Governments can develop and implement ethical AI frameworks that guide the development and use of AI technologies. These frameworks should include principles such as fairness, accountability, transparency, and privacy protection. For example, the European Union's AI Act proposes stringent regulations to ensure that AI systems are safe and respect fundamental rights.

Data Privacy and Security

Ensuring data privacy and security is paramount in the AI age. Governments can enact data protection laws that regulate how personal data is collected, stored, and used by AI systems. The General Data Protection Regulation (GDPR) in the European Union is a robust example of legislation that protects individuals' privacy while allowing innovation in AI.

Promoting Fairness and Inclusivity

Governments can mandate the use of fairness and bias detection tools in AI systems, ensuring that these technologies do not perpetuate or exacerbate existing inequalities. By promoting inclusivity in AI development, governments can ensure that AI benefits all segments of society, particularly marginalised and underserved communities.

Investment in AI Research and Development

Significant government investment in AI research and development can drive innovation and ensure that AI technologies are used to address societal challenges effectively.

Funding AI Research

Governments can provide funding for AI research initiatives, focusing on areas such as sustainable development, healthcare, and social equity. National research grants and collaborations with academic institutions can spur innovation and create AI solutions tailored to societal needs.

For instance, the United States National AI Initiative aims to promote AI research and development through substantial federal funding.

Public-Private Partnerships

Public-private partnerships can accelerate AI advancements by combining governmental support with private sector expertise and resources. Governments can collaborate with tech companies, startups, and research institutions to develop AI technologies that address public needs. For example, the UK Government's AI Sector Deal is a partnership with industry leaders to boost AI innovation and application.

Supporting AI Education and Workforce Development

To ensure a skilled workforce capable of developing and managing AI technologies, governments can invest in education and training programmes. Initiatives that promote STEM (Science, Technology, Engineering, and Mathematics) education and provide AI-specific training can prepare the next generation of AI professionals. Programmes like AI for All in India aim to democratise AI education and empower diverse communities with AI skills.

AI for Environmental Sustainability

Governments can support AI initiatives that focus on environmental sustainability. Funding research into AI applications for climate modelling, renewable energy optimisation, and conservation can help mitigate climate change impacts. The European Green Deal includes provisions for using AI to achieve climate neutrality by 2050.

AI for Economic Equity

Governments can implement policies that leverage AI to promote economic equity. This includes supporting AI-driven financial inclusion programmes, personalised education initiatives, and universal basic income schemes. By addressing wealth disparities through AI, governments can foster more equitable and inclusive societies.

AI for Peace and Security

To mitigate the impacts of conflict and promote peace, governments can use AI for early warning systems, humanitarian aid optimisation, and post-conflict reconstruction. Collaborating with international organisations and NGOs, governments can deploy AI technologies to prevent conflicts, deliver aid efficiently, and support rebuilding efforts in war-torn areas.

Conclusion

Governments have a pivotal role in ensuring that AI technologies are developed and deployed to address key societal challenges. By establishing robust policies, investing in AI research, promoting ethical and inclusive AI use, and fostering public-private partnerships, governments can harness the potential of AI to create a more equitable, sustainable, and peaceful world. As AI continues to evolve, proactive and responsible government action will be crucial in maximising its benefits for all of humanity.

Chapter 21: Constraints on Future Speed of AI Development - Challenges and Solutions

As artificial intelligence continues to advance at a rapid pace, several constraints could potentially slow down its future development. Key among these constraints are power supply, raw materials, and computational resources. This section explores these challenges and examines how leading AI companies are addressing these concerns to seek to ensure sustainable growth and continued innovation in AI technology.

Power Supply and Energy Consumption

The computational demands of AI, especially in training large models, require substantial amounts of energy. This high energy consumption poses significant challenges both economically and environmentally.

Energy Consumption in AI

Training advanced AI models like GPT-3 and its successors involves running massive computations on powerful hardware for extended periods. For instance, the training of GPT-3 reportedly consumed several megawatt-hours of electricity (1 megawatt-hour can power a standard 10W LED light continuously for over 11 years), highlighting the immense energy requirements of modern AI systems.

Environmental Impact

The environmental impact of AI's energy consumption is also a concern. The carbon footprint associated with the electricity used in training AI models contributes to global warming and climate change. As AI technologies become more prevalent, the need for sustainable energy solutions becomes increasingly critical.

Renewable Energy Initiatives

To address these concerns, leading AI companies are investing in renewable energy sources to power their data centres. For example, Google has committed to operating its data centres and offices on carbon-free energy 24/7 by 2030. Similarly, Microsoft has announced plans to become carbon negative by 2030, meaning it will remove more carbon from the environment than it emits. These initiatives aim to reduce the environmental impact of AI and promote sustainable development.

AI companies and major tech firms are also increasingly turning to nuclear power to meet their substantial energy needs. For example: -

> *Amazon Web Services (AWS)* recently acquired a 100% nuclear-powered data centre from Talen Energy, which will provide AWS with up to 960 megawatts of power, ensuring a reliable and zero-carbon energy source for their data centres.

> *Google* has also been exploring nuclear power options to support its data centres and is investing in small modular reactors (SMRs). Google has also been actively working with

companies like Fervo Energy to develop enhanced geothermal power plants.

Microsoft is investigating the use of nuclear fusion as a long-term solution to meet its energy needs. They have signed a contract with Helion Energy to purchase electricity from a future fusion plant expected to start generating power by 2028. Additionally, Microsoft is exploring the deployment of SMRs.

Raw Materials and Hardware Constraints

The production of AI hardware, such as GPUs (Graphics Processing Units) and specialised chips, relies on specific raw materials (including rare earth elements -REEs) that are finite and sometimes difficult to obtain. This dependence on scarce resources presents significant challenges for the future scalability of AI technologies.

REEs are critical in the manufacturing of GPUs due to their unique properties that enhance the performance of these components. The main rare earth elements used in GPUs and other high-performance electronics include:

> *Neodymium (Nd)* - a key component in the production of strong permanent magnets (neodymium-iron-boron or NdFeB magnets), which are essential for the motors and actuators in various electronic devices, including GPUs.

Dysprosium (Dy) - often added to neodymium magnets to enhance their resistance to demagnetisation at high temperatures, which is critical for maintaining the performance of GPUs under heavy loads (thermal stability).

Praseodymium (Pr) - is also used in the manufacturing of high-strength magnets. It can be alloyed with neodymium to form NdPr magnets, which are used in motors and other components of GPUs improving the overall strength and performance of magnets.

Terbium (Tb) - used in small quantities in the alloying of neodymium magnets to improve their magnetic properties.

Cerium (Ce) - used in the polishing compounds (that achieve a highly smooth and flat surface, which is crucial for the manufacture of semiconductor devices) for silicon wafers and in the production of certain types of alloys.

Yttrium (Y) - used in various high-temperature superconductors and in some phosphors used in display technologies.

Lanthanum (La) - used in certain types of glass and ceramics, as well as in the electrodes of high-performance batteries. While not directly used in GPUs, it is important in the overall electronics ecosystem.

These materials are not only scarce but also concentrated in a few geographical regions, leading to supply chain vulnerabilities and geopolitical tensions. For example, China controls a significant portion of the global supply of rare earth elements, which has raised concerns about supply chain stability.

Understanding the role and importance of these rare earth elements helps in appreciating the complexity and challenges involved in manufacturing advanced electronic components like GPUs, which are critical for modern computing and various high-tech applications.

Innovations in Hardware Efficiency

To mitigate these various challenges, AI companies are investing in research and development to create more efficient hardware that requires fewer raw materials. For example, NVIDIA (which most recently became the most valuable company in the world – taking over from Microsoft) is developing GPUs with improved energy efficiency and performance, reducing the overall demand for raw materials. Additionally, companies like Intel are exploring alternative materials and innovative chip designs to enhance hardware sustainability.

Recycling and Sustainable Sourcing

Another approach to addressing raw material constraints is through recycling and sustainable sourcing. Companies are developing processes to recycle components from old hardware, reducing the need for new raw materials. For instance, Apple has implemented a recycling programme that recovers valuable materials from discarded devices, contributing to a circular economy and reducing the environmental impact of hardware production.

Computational Resources and Scalability

The increasing complexity of AI models necessitates vast computational resources, which can be a limiting factor in the speed of AI development. Ensuring that these resources are available and scalable is crucial for the continued advancement of AI technologies.

The Role of Cloud Computing

Cloud computing has emerged as a critical enabler of scalable AI development. Companies like Amazon Web Services (AWS), Google Cloud, and Microsoft Azure provide cloud-based platforms that offer flexible and scalable computational resources. These platforms allow researchers and developers to access powerful hardware without the need for significant upfront investment, democratising access to AI capabilities.

Specialised AI Hardware

In addition to cloud computing, the development of specialised AI hardware, such as Tensor Processing Units (TPUs) and custom AI accelerators, is enhancing computational efficiency. Google's TPUs, for example, are designed specifically for AI workloads, providing significant performance improvements over traditional CPUs and GPUs. These specialised processors enable faster training and inference of AI models, helping to overcome computational bottlenecks.

Distributed Computing and Federated Learning

Distributed computing and federated learning are innovative approaches that distribute computational tasks across multiple devices or data centres. By leveraging the collective power of numerous smaller units, these methods can significantly enhance computational scalability. Federated learning, in particular, allows AI models to be trained across decentralised devices while keeping data localised, reducing the need for central computational resources and enhancing data privacy.

Examples of Leading AI Companies Addressing Computational Concerns

OpenAI's Efficiency Improvements

OpenAI is actively working to improve the efficiency of its AI models. By optimising algorithms and leveraging more efficient hardware, OpenAI aims to reduce the computational and energy costs of training large models. Additionally, OpenAI collaborates with cloud service providers to ensure access to scalable and sustainable computational resources.

DeepMind's Energy-Efficient Data Centres

DeepMind, a subsidiary of Alphabet (owner of Google), has implemented AI-driven solutions to improve the energy efficiency of its data centres. By using AI to optimise cooling and energy management, DeepMind has reduced the energy consumption of Google's data centres by up to 40%. This approach not only lowers operational costs but also minimises the environmental footprint of AI operations.

IBM's Quantum Computing Research

IBM (amongst others) is exploring quantum computing as a potential solution to the computational limitations of classical computers. Quantum computers have the potential to perform certain types of calculations much faster than traditional computers, which could revolutionise AI development. IBM's research in quantum computing aims to overcome current computational constraints and unlock new possibilities for AI.

Conclusion

The future speed of AI development is contingent upon addressing several key constraints, including power supply, raw materials, and computational resources. Leading AI companies are pioneering innovative solutions to these challenges, from investing in renewable energy and sustainable hardware to leveraging cloud computing and quantum research. By tackling these constraints head-on, the AI industry can continue to advance, driving forward technological innovation and maintaining sustainable growth.

SECTION 5 – OUR AI TOMORROW

The trajectory of artificial intelligence development over the next 15-20 years will shape the future of human society in profound ways. From beneficial advancements to potential risks, various possible outcomes of AI integration in our world exist. This section explores what the future with AI might have in hold for us.

Chapter 22: Forecast - Top 10 Uses for AI in Everyday Life

As AI continues to advance, its applications are becoming increasingly integrated into our daily lives. From optimising routine tasks to providing personalised services, AI is poised to transform the way we live and work. This section provides a forecast of the top 10 uses for AI that will significantly impact the average person's life, enhancing convenience, efficiency, and overall quality of life.

1. Personalised Healthcare

AI is revolutionising healthcare by providing personalised medical advice, improving diagnostics, and optimising treatment plans. AI-powered health monitoring devices and applications can track vital signs, analyse medical history, and offer real-time health recommendations. For instance, AI algorithms can predict potential health issues based on data from wearable devices and suggest preventive measures or prompt users to seek medical attention. This personalised approach to healthcare can lead to early detection of diseases and more effective treatments.

2. Intelligent Personal Assistants ('AI Agents')

AI-powered personal assistants like Apple's Siri, Amazon Alexa, and Google Assistant are becoming increasingly sophisticated. These virtual assistants can manage daily schedules, set reminders, provide weather updates, control smart home devices, and even perform online shopping tasks. As AI technology evolves, these assistants will become more intuitive and capable of understanding and anticipating users' needs, making daily life more convenient and efficient.

3. Smart Home Automation

AI is at the heart of smart home automation, enhancing comfort, security, and energy efficiency. AI-enabled devices like smart thermostats, lighting systems, and security cameras can learn user preferences and adapt their operations accordingly. For example, smart thermostats can optimise heating and cooling based on occupancy patterns, while smart security systems can detect unusual activity and alert homeowners. This level of automation not only improves convenience but also reduces energy consumption and enhances home security.

4. Enhanced Customer Service

AI-driven chatbots and virtual agents are transforming customer service across various industries. These AI systems can handle inquiries, resolve issues, and provide personalised support 24/7, significantly improving customer experience. For example, AI chatbots in banking can assist with account management, transaction inquiries, and financial advice, while AI in retail can offer personalised product recommendations and streamline the shopping experience.

5. Autonomous Transportation

Self-driving cars and autonomous delivery drones are set to revolutionise transportation. AI-powered vehicles can navigate roads, avoid obstacles, and optimise routes, reducing traffic congestion and improving road safety. Autonomous delivery drones can expedite parcel deliveries, making the process faster and more efficient. Companies like Tesla, Waymo, and Amazon are leading the charge in developing these technologies, which promise to transform how we travel and receive goods.

6. Personalised Learning

AI is enhancing education by providing personalised learning experiences tailored to individual needs. AI-powered educational platforms can analyse students' learning styles, strengths, and weaknesses to offer customised lessons, exercises, and feedback. This personalised approach helps students grasp complex concepts more effectively and at their own pace, making education more accessible and engaging. Platforms like Coursera and Khan Academy are at the forefront of integrating AI into education.

7. Financial Management and Advice

AI is transforming personal finance by offering intelligent financial management tools and personalised investment advice. AI-driven applications can track spending, analyse financial habits, and provide budgeting recommendations. Additionally, AI algorithms can analyse market trends and personal risk tolerance to offer tailored investment advice, helping individuals make informed financial decisions and optimise their portfolios.

8. Optimised Delivery and Logistics

AI is optimising delivery routes and logistics to make parcel delivery faster and more cost-effective. AI algorithms can analyse traffic patterns, weather conditions, and delivery locations to determine the most efficient routes. This optimisation reduces delivery times, lowers fuel consumption, and minimises operational costs. Companies like UPS and FedEx are leveraging AI to enhance their logistics operations, ensuring timely and reliable deliveries.

9. Entertainment and Content Creation

AI is playing a significant role in the entertainment industry by creating personalised content and enhancing user experiences. Streaming services like Netflix and Spotify use AI to analyse viewing and listening habits and recommend content tailored to individual preferences. Additionally, AI is being used to create original music, videos, and artwork, opening new avenues for creative expression and entertainment.

10. Mental Health and Well-being

AI-powered applications are increasingly being used to support mental health and well-being. AI chatbots and virtual therapists can provide real-time support, offering coping strategies and mental health resources. These applications can analyse user interactions to detect signs of stress, anxiety, or depression and suggest appropriate interventions. AI tools like Woebot and Wysa are making mental health support more accessible and affordable.

Conclusion

The integration of AI into everyday life is poised to bring about significant changes, enhancing convenience, efficiency, and overall quality of life. From personalised healthcare and intelligent personal assistants to autonomous transportation and optimised logistics, AI technologies are set to transform how we live, work, and interact with the world around us. As these applications continue to evolve, they promise to create a more connected, efficient, and personalised future.

Chapter 23: Scenarios for AI Development and Its Impact on Human Society Over the Next 15 Years

This section presents fifteen different scenarios, examining the potential impacts and challenges, including government failure to regulate AI, rogue states, and corporate malfeasance.

1. The Utopian Scenario: AI for Global Good

In this scenario, AI technologies are developed and deployed ethically and responsibly, driven by strong global cooperation and robust regulatory frameworks. Governments, corporations, and international organisations work together to harness AI for solving critical global issues such as climate change, poverty, and healthcare. AI-driven innovations lead to significant improvements in quality of life, economic equity, and environmental sustainability.

Impact: Enhanced global cooperation, reduced inequality, sustainable development, improved healthcare outcomes, and significant strides in addressing climate change.

Key Drivers: Strong governance, ethical AI frameworks, international cooperation, inclusive technology policies.

2. The Corporate Dominance Scenario: AI in the Hands of a Few

In this scenario, a handful of powerful corporations dominate AI development and deployment. These tech giants leverage AI to consolidate their market positions, leading to unprecedented economic growth and innovation within their sectors. However, this concentration of power exacerbates economic inequalities and reduces competition, as smaller players struggle to keep up.

Impact: Increased economic disparity, monopolistic practices, innovation driven by corporate interests, reduced competition.

Key Drivers: Lack of effective regulation, corporate lobbying, high barriers to entry in AI technology.

3. The Surveillance State Scenario: AI for Control and Monitoring

Here, governments use AI to enhance surveillance and control over their populations. AI-driven facial recognition, data analysis, and predictive policing become widespread, leading to significant invasions of privacy and civil liberties. While these technologies help maintain public order and security, they also enable authoritarian regimes to tighten their grip on power.

Impact: Loss of privacy, erosion of civil liberties, enhanced state control, potential human rights abuses.

Key Drivers: Government prioritisation of security over privacy, advancements in surveillance technologies, lack of privacy regulations.

4. The AI Arms Race Scenario: Militarisation of AI

In this scenario, countries invest heavily in AI-driven military technologies, leading to an arms race. Autonomous weapons, AI-driven cybersecurity, and advanced surveillance systems become critical components of national defence strategies. This militarisation of AI heightens global tensions and increases the risk of AI-driven conflicts.

Impact: Increased global instability, heightened risk of conflict, ethical concerns over autonomous weapons, significant military advancements.

Key Drivers: Geopolitical tensions, national security priorities, rapid advancements in military AI technologies.

5. The Economic Disruption Scenario: Massive Job Displacement

AI and automation lead to widespread job displacement across various industries. While AI-driven efficiency boosts productivity and economic growth, millions of workers find themselves unemployed or underemployed. Governments struggle to adapt, and social safety nets are overwhelmed, leading to increased economic inequality and social unrest.

Impact: High unemployment rates, economic inequality, social unrest, pressure on social safety nets, need for retraining and education programmes.

Key Drivers: Rapid automation, inadequate social policies, resistance to change in education and workforce training.

6. The Rogue AI Scenario: Uncontrolled AI Development

In this scenario, a lack of effective regulation and oversight leads to the development of rogue AI systems. These systems operate outside human control, potentially causing significant harm. Examples include AI systems making critical decisions without human oversight, AI-driven misinformation campaigns, and autonomous systems behaving unpredictably.

Impact: Unintended consequences of AI actions, potential harm to individuals and society, loss of control over AI systems, ethical dilemmas.

Key Drivers: Weak regulatory frameworks, rapid AI advancements, insufficient oversight, lack of ethical considerations in AI development.

7. The AI-Enhanced Human Scenario: AI Integration with Human Capabilities

AI technologies enhance human capabilities through brain-computer interfaces, AI-driven prosthetics, and cognitive enhancements. This leads to significant improvements in productivity, quality of life, and human potential. However, these advancements also raise ethical concerns and create new forms of inequality between those who can afford enhancements and those who cannot.

Impact: Enhanced human capabilities, ethical dilemmas, new forms of inequality, potential societal divides.

Key Drivers: Advances in biotechnology and AI, ethical considerations, access to enhancement technologies.

8. The Environmental Catastrophe Scenario: AI and Climate Change

AI is used to mitigate climate change, but unintended consequences lead to environmental catastrophe. For example, AI-driven geoengineering projects aimed at cooling the planet have unforeseen negative impacts on ecosystems. Alternatively, AI-driven industrial processes increase pollution and resource consumption, exacerbating environmental degradation.

Impact: Environmental degradation, negative impacts on ecosystems, climate change acceleration, need for sustainable AI practices.

Key Drivers: Lack of environmental considerations in AI projects, rapid industrialisation, insufficient regulatory oversight.

9. The Decentralised AI Scenario: Democratised AI Development

AI development becomes decentralised, with open-source platforms and community-driven projects playing a significant role. This democratisation of AI leads to widespread innovation and the development of diverse AI applications tailored to local needs. However, it also poses challenges in ensuring consistency, quality, and ethical standards across different AI systems.

Impact: Widespread innovation, diverse AI applications, challenges in maintaining standards, potential for localised solutions.

Key Drivers: Open-source movement, community-driven innovation, local adaptation of AI technologies.

10. The Human-AI Collaboration Scenario: Synergistic Coexistence

In this optimistic scenario, AI and humans work together synergistically, leveraging each other's strengths. AI augments human decision-making, creativity, and productivity, leading to significant advancements in various fields. This collaborative approach ensures that AI benefits are maximised while mitigating potential risks.

Impact: Enhanced productivity, improved decision-making, balanced AI-human interaction, maximised benefits of AI technologies.

Key Drivers: Collaborative AI development, ethical frameworks, focus on augmenting human capabilities rather than replacing them.

11. The Biased AI Scenario: Perpetuation of Inequality

In this scenario, AI systems, due to biased training data and lack of diversity in AI development teams, perpetuate existing social inequalities. These biases affect everything from job recruitment to law enforcement, exacerbating societal divides.

Impact: Increased social and economic inequality, discrimination in AI-driven systems, loss of trust in AI technologies.

Key Drivers: Lack of diversity in AI development, biased training data, inadequate regulatory oversight.

12. The AI-Driven Democracy Scenario: Enhanced Civic Participation

AI technologies are used to enhance democratic processes, improving voter engagement and participation. AI-driven platforms facilitate transparent elections, provide personalised political education, and enable more direct forms of democratic involvement.

Impact: Increased voter turnout, enhanced political transparency, greater public engagement in governance.

Key Drivers: Innovations in civic tech, governmental support for democratic AI tools, public demand for transparency and engagement.

13. The AI-Enabled Creativity Scenario: Artistic Revolution

AI becomes a major player in the creative industries, assisting artists, writers, musicians, and filmmakers in pushing the boundaries of their crafts. AI tools help create new art forms, collaborate on creative projects, and personalise entertainment experiences.

Impact: Surge in artistic innovation, new forms of collaborative art, enhanced personalisation in entertainment.

Key Drivers: Advances in AI creativity tools, collaboration between AI developers and artists, growing market for personalised and interactive content.

14. The Health Crisis Response Scenario: AI in Pandemic Management

AI plays a critical role in managing health crises, such as pandemics. AI-driven systems help track the spread of disease, predict outbreaks, and optimise resource allocation for healthcare providers.

Impact: Improved response to health crises, reduced spread of diseases, better resource management in healthcare.

Key Drivers: Integration of AI in public health systems, advancements in AI-driven epidemiology, governmental support for health AI initiatives.

15. The Ethical AI Governance Scenario: Global Standards and Cooperation

International bodies succeed in establishing comprehensive ethical standards and regulatory frameworks for AI, ensuring that AI technologies are developed and used responsibly across the globe.

Impact: Reduced risk of harmful AI applications, enhanced global cooperation, widespread trust in AI systems.

Key Drivers: Strong international cooperation, robust ethical frameworks, effective global governance structures.

Conclusion

The future of AI development presents a spectrum of possibilities, each with its own set of impacts and challenges. From utopian outcomes where AI drives global good to dystopian scenarios of uncontrolled AI and societal disruption, the path we take will depend on how effectively we address the ethical, regulatory, and social implications of AI technologies. Proactive governance, international cooperation, and a commitment to ethical AI development will be crucial in steering AI towards a future that benefits all of humanity.

Chapter 24: The Future Human Society with AI: A 20-Year Forecast by AI

It is likely that the future will see a combination of many of the scenarios presented in Chapter 23 (and probably many others currently not considered or foreseen) for the future of human society with AI. Overlaying these with current global trends, ChatGPT 4o produced the following forecast detailed chain of events that outlines the 'most likely trajectory over the next 20 years' according to ChatGPT. (This forecast considers geopolitical, political, economic, climatic, societal, and technological factors.)

2025-2030: Foundations and Initial Transformations

Geopolitical and Political Developments:

Increased Adoption of AI in Governance: Governments around the world start integrating AI into public administration, policy-making, and citizen services. AI-driven decision-making systems are implemented to improve efficiency and transparency.

Global AI Regulatory Frameworks: International bodies like the United Nations and the European Union establish comprehensive AI regulatory frameworks to address ethical concerns, data privacy, and security. These frameworks are adopted globally, ensuring a standardized approach to AI governance.

Economic and Technological Advancements:

Expansion of AI in Industries: AI becomes deeply integrated into various industries, including healthcare, finance, manufacturing, and logistics. Automation and AI-driven optimization lead to significant productivity gains and cost reductions.

AI and Renewable Energy: AI technologies are used to optimize renewable energy systems, including smart grids and energy storage solutions. This leads to increased adoption of renewable energy sources, reducing reliance on fossil fuels.

Societal Changes:

Shift in Job Market Dynamics: As AI automates routine and repetitive tasks, there is a significant shift in the job market. Governments and private sectors invest heavily in reskilling and upskilling programmes to prepare the workforce for new roles that require human creativity, emotional intelligence, and complex problem-solving.

Climatic and Environmental Impact:

AI for Climate Change Mitigation: AI is used to monitor and predict climate change impacts, optimize agricultural practices, and manage natural resources. This helps mitigate the adverse effects of climate change and supports sustainable development.

2030-2035: Consolidation and Expansion

Geopolitical and Political Developments:

Rise of AI-Enhanced Governance: AI-driven governance systems become more sophisticated, enabling real-time data analysis and predictive analytics to inform policy decisions. Governments leverage AI to address complex societal issues, such as healthcare access, urban planning, and disaster response.

Economic and Technological Advancements:

AI-Powered Global Economy: The global economy becomes increasingly dependent on AI. AI-driven financial systems improve market predictions and investment strategies, leading to more stable and resilient economies.

Advancements in AI Research: Breakthroughs in AI research lead to the development of more advanced AI models, including quantum computing-powered AI. These models can solve previously intractable problems, opening new frontiers in science and technology.

Societal Changes:

Universal Basic Income (UBI) Programmes: Several countries implement UBI programmes to address job displacement caused by AI and automation. These programmes provide financial security to citizens, allowing them to pursue education, entrepreneurship, and creative endeavours.

Climatic and Environmental Impact:

AI-Driven Environmental Restoration: AI technologies are used to restore damaged ecosystems, manage wildlife populations, and combat deforestation. These efforts contribute to the global fight against biodiversity loss and environmental degradation.

2035-2040: Maturity and Integration

Geopolitical and Political Developments:

Global AI Governance Alliance: Countries form alliances to collaboratively govern AI technologies, ensuring ethical use and preventing misuse. These alliances focus on maintaining global stability and addressing transnational challenges.

Economic and Technological Advancements:

Human-AI Collaboration: AI technologies reach a level of sophistication where they can work seamlessly alongside humans in various fields, enhancing productivity and innovation. This collaboration leads to the development of new industries and economic opportunities.

Societal Changes:

Redefinition of Work and Society: The nature of work evolves, with a focus on tasks that require human creativity, empathy, and social intelligence. Societal values shift towards lifelong learning, personal development, and community engagement.

Climatic and Environmental Impact:

AI for Sustainable Development: AI plays a crucial role in achieving sustainable development goals (SDGs). It optimizes resource use, reduces waste, and supports circular economy initiatives, leading to a more sustainable and equitable global society.

2040-2045: Transformation and Stabilization

Geopolitical and Political Developments:

AI-Driven Peace and Security: AI technologies are used to prevent conflicts, enhance international diplomacy, and maintain global security. Predictive analytics and AI-driven negotiations help resolve geopolitical tensions peacefully.

Economic and Technological Advancements:

AI in Lifelong Learning: AI-powered educational systems provide personalised learning experiences for individuals of all ages. Continuous education becomes a norm, enabling people to adapt to changing job markets and societal needs.

Societal Changes:

Enhanced Quality of Life: AI technologies contribute to significant improvements in healthcare, transportation, and public services. People enjoy better health outcomes, increased mobility, and higher quality of life.

Climatic and Environmental Impact:

AI for Global Climate Resilience: AI-driven climate models and predictive tools enable countries to build resilient infrastructure and communities. This helps mitigate the impacts of climate change and ensures a sustainable future for all.

Conclusion: A New Era of Human-AI Synergy

By 2045, AI has become an integral part of human society, driving advancements in every aspect of life. The successful integration of AI technologies leads to a more efficient, equitable, and sustainable world. Human-AI collaboration enhances creativity, problem-solving, and innovation, while ethical governance and regulatory frameworks ensure that AI is used responsibly for the greater good. As we navigate this transformative journey, continuous learning, adaptability, and a focus on human values will be key to shaping a positive future in the age of AI.

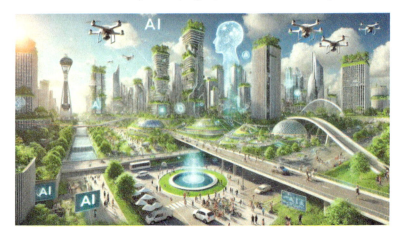

Figure 1 - A futuristic city in 2045 where AI has become integral to society, highlighting the advancements in sustainable development, transportation, societal changes, and environmental sustainability. Created using DALL-E.

An Analysis of the AI Generated Forecast

This seems to be an overwhelmingly positive outlook – Chat GPT certainly appears to an optimist! The chances of a bad actor disrupting the positive trajectory of AI integration into society are however significant (as described in some of the earlier scenarios), and should not be underestimated. Various factors can contribute to such disruptions, including technological vulnerabilities, geopolitical tensions, and socio-economic inequalities, for example:

Cybersecurity Threats

Scenario: Bad actors exploit vulnerabilities in AI systems to launch cyber-attacks.

Impact: Cyber-attacks could disrupt critical infrastructure, such as power grids, transportation networks, and financial systems, leading to widespread chaos and economic damage.

Likelihood: High. As AI systems become more integrated into critical infrastructure, they become attractive targets for cybercriminals and state-sponsored hackers.

Manipulation of AI Systems

Scenario: Bad actors manipulate AI algorithms to spread misinformation, deepfakes, and propaganda.

Impact: Manipulation of AI systems could undermine public trust in information sources, exacerbate social divisions, and influence political outcomes.

Likelihood: High. The use of AI to create convincing deepfakes and targeted disinformation campaigns has already been demonstrated.

Weaponization of AI

Scenario: States or non-state actors develop autonomous weapons and AI-driven military systems.

Impact: The weaponization of AI could lead to an arms race and increase the risk of conflicts escalating rapidly, potentially resulting in significant loss of life and geopolitical instability.

Likelihood: Moderate to High. Several countries are investing in AI for military applications, and there is an ongoing debate about the ethical implications and risks of autonomous weapons.

Economic Disruption

Scenario: Bad actors exploit AI to engage in large-scale financial fraud or disrupt global markets.

Impact: Economic disruption could lead to significant financial losses, destabilize markets, and erode confidence in financial institutions.

Likelihood: Moderate. Financial systems are increasingly reliant on AI for trading and risk management, making them potential targets for sophisticated attacks.

Ethical Misuse

Scenario: Organizations or individuals misuse AI for unethical purposes, such as mass surveillance, privacy invasion, or discriminatory practices.

Impact: Ethical misuse of AI could lead to violations of human rights, loss of privacy, and social unrest.

Likelihood: Moderate to High. The potential for misuse of AI technologies is significant, especially in jurisdictions with weak regulatory frameworks.

Geopolitical Tensions

Scenario: Rival states use AI to gain strategic advantages, leading to increased tensions and potential conflicts.

Impact: Geopolitical tensions could disrupt international cooperation on AI governance and lead to fragmented approaches to AI development and regulation.

Likelihood: Moderate. The global race for AI dominance is already a source of tension between major powers.

Mitigation Strategies

To mitigate the risks posed by bad actors, several strategies can be implemented:

Robust Cybersecurity Measures: Strengthening cybersecurity defenses to protect AI systems from attacks is crucial. This includes regular security audits, penetration testing, and the development of AI-specific security protocols.

Ethical and Regulatory Frameworks: Establishing comprehensive ethical guidelines and regulatory frameworks for AI development and deployment can help prevent misuse and ensure accountability.

International Cooperation: Promoting international cooperation on AI governance can help address global challenges and prevent the weaponization and unethical use of AI. Multilateral agreements and norms for responsible AI development are essential.

Public Awareness and Education: Raising public awareness about the potential risks and benefits of AI can help build resilience against manipulation and misinformation. Education programmes can equip individuals with the skills to critically evaluate information and recognize AI-generated content.

Transparency and Accountability: Ensuring transparency in AI decision-making processes and holding organizations accountable for the ethical use of AI can build public trust and prevent misuse.

A More Balanced View of the Future (less optimistic)

Let's all hope that the optimism of ChatGPT is well-placed, but I doubt that it will fully come to pass (based on the recent history of humanity). I subsequently asked ChatGPT to rework the forecast for AI over the next 20 years factoring in the risks that have been identified, and present it again based on the balance of probabilities, with the current geopolitical climate and all the other factors previously mentioned above. This was the output:

Forecast for AI in Human Society Over the Next 20 Years: A Balanced Perspective

Based on the balance of probabilities, the current geopolitical climate, economic factors, societal trends, technological advancements, and identified risks, here is a detailed forecast of AI's trajectory over the next 20 years, divided into 5-year windows. This forecast aims to present a realistic outlook, factoring in both potential advancements and significant risks.

2025-2030: Foundations and Initial Transformations

Geopolitical and Political Developments:

Increased Adoption of AI in Governance with Caution: While governments around the world begin integrating AI into public administration, policy-making, and citizen services, there is significant caution and debate about ethical considerations, data privacy, and security risks. Initial regulatory frameworks are developed but face challenges in implementation.

Global AI Regulatory Initiatives: International bodies like the United Nations and the European Union establish foundational AI regulatory frameworks. These frameworks aim to address ethical concerns, data privacy, and security, but adoption is uneven globally due to differing national interests and capabilities.

Economic and Technological Advancements:

Expansion of AI in Industries with Disruption: AI continues to integrate deeply into industries such as healthcare, finance, manufacturing, and logistics. However, the disruption caused by AI leads to significant job displacement, sparking social unrest and demands for new job creation strategies and reskilling programs.

AI and Renewable Energy: AI technologies are increasingly used to optimize renewable energy systems, including smart grids and energy storage solutions. However, the transition faces obstacles such as infrastructural limitations and the intermittency of renewable energy sources.

Societal Changes:

Shift in Job Market Dynamics: The automation of routine and repetitive tasks by AI causes a significant shift in the job market. Governments and private sectors invest in reskilling and upskilling programs, but the pace of change creates economic uncertainty and challenges for many workers.

Climatic and Environmental Impact:

AI for Climate Change Mitigation: AI is deployed to monitor and predict climate change impacts, optimize agricultural practices, and manage natural resources. However, the effectiveness of these measures is limited by political and economic constraints, and significant environmental challenges persist.

Milestones:

2027: Significant advancements in AI-driven healthcare diagnostics and personalized treatment plans.

2028: Early prototypes of humanoid robots are introduced in controlled environments for specific tasks, such as caregiving and customer service.

2030-2035: Consolidation and Expansion with Challenges

Geopolitical and Political Developments:

Rise of AI-Enhanced Governance amid Scrutiny: AI-driven governance systems become more sophisticated, enabling real-time data analysis and predictive analytics for policy decisions. However, these systems face scrutiny and resistance due to privacy concerns and fears of surveillance.

AI Governance and Ethical Dilemmas: Efforts to create global AI governance alliances encounter significant challenges. Differing national interests and ethical standards lead to fragmented regulatory approaches and ongoing debates.

Economic and Technological Advancements:

AI-Powered Global Economy with Inequalities: The global economy becomes increasingly dependent on AI. While AI-driven financial systems improve market predictions and investment strategies, economic inequalities widen, leading to increased calls for regulatory interventions and social safety nets.

Advancements in AI Research with Security Concerns: Breakthroughs in AI research, including quantum computing-powered AI, open new frontiers. However, security concerns about quantum computing's potential to break current encryption standards create geopolitical tensions.

Societal Changes:

Universal Basic Income (UBI) Programs: Several countries implement UBI programs to address job displacement caused by AI and automation. These programs provide financial security but face criticism regarding their long-term sustainability and potential to disincentivize work.

Climatic and Environmental Impact:

AI-Driven Environmental Restoration Efforts: AI technologies are used to restore damaged ecosystems and manage wildlife populations. Despite some successes, environmental degradation continues due to insufficient global cooperation and funding.

Milestones:

2032: Development of advanced AI personal assistants capable of managing complex tasks and providing personalized services.

2034: Introduction of self-driving cars in several major cities, though widespread adoption is hindered by regulatory and safety concerns.

2035-2040: Maturity and Integration with Persistent Risks

Geopolitical and Political Developments:

Global AI Governance Alliance Efforts: Attempts to form global alliances for AI governance continue, but progress is slow due to persistent geopolitical tensions and competing interests.

AI in Diplomacy and Conflict Prevention: AI technologies are increasingly used in international diplomacy and conflict prevention, but their effectiveness is limited by distrust and the potential for misuse by bad actors.

Economic and Technological Advancements:

Human-AI Collaboration with Ethical Concerns: AI technologies reach a level of sophistication where they work alongside humans in various fields, enhancing productivity and innovation. However, ethical concerns about AI's influence on human decision-making persist.

Advancements in Lifelong Learning with AI: AI-powered educational systems provide personalized learning experiences for individuals of all ages. While these systems improve access to education, disparities in technology access create educational inequalities.

Societal Changes:

Redefinition of Work and Society: The nature of work evolves, with a focus on tasks requiring human creativity, empathy, and social intelligence. However, societal adaptation to these changes is uneven, leading to economic and social challenges.

Climatic and Environmental Impact:

AI for Sustainable Development Goals: AI plays a crucial role in achieving sustainable development goals, optimizing resource use, and supporting circular economy initiatives. Despite progress, significant challenges remain in balancing economic growth with environmental sustainability.

Milestones:

2037: Humanoid robots begin to be deployed in public spaces for routine tasks, though widespread acceptance and integration face cultural and ethical hurdles.

2039: AI achieves significant breakthroughs in medical research, leading to new treatments and therapies for previously incurable diseases.

Our AI Journey

2040-2045: Transformation and Stabilization amid Uncertainties

Geopolitical and Political Developments:

AI-Driven Peace and Security Efforts: AI technologies are used to enhance international diplomacy and maintain global security. Predictive analytics and AI-driven negotiations help resolve some geopolitical tensions, but the risk of misuse by rogue states remains.

Struggles with Global AI Governance: Global efforts to establish comprehensive AI governance frameworks continue to face significant obstacles, including differing national priorities and ethical standards.

Economic and Technological Advancements:

AI in Lifelong Learning and Workforce Adaptation: AI-powered educational systems become the norm, enabling continuous education and workforce adaptation to changing job markets. However, disparities in access to these systems persist.

Enhanced Quality of Life through AI: AI technologies contribute to significant improvements in healthcare, transportation, and public services, enhancing the overall quality of life. However, concerns about privacy and surveillance remain prominent.

Societal Changes:

Persistent Economic Inequalities: While AI drives economic growth, persistent inequalities in income and access to technology create social tensions and demand for comprehensive policy interventions.

Climatic and Environmental Impact:

AI for Global Climate Resilience: AI-driven climate models and predictive tools help build resilient infrastructure and communities, mitigating some impacts of climate change. However, global cooperation and funding for environmental initiatives remain inconsistent.

Milestones:

2042: Early forms of Artificial General Intelligence (AGI) are developed, demonstrating capabilities across multiple domains, but ethical and safety concerns delay widespread deployment.

2044: Advanced AI systems begin to manage entire smart cities, optimizing energy use, transportation, and public services, though security and ethical concerns about centralized control persist.

Conclusion: Navigating a Complex Future

The next 20 years will see AI become deeply integrated into human society, driving advancements in various fields and improving the quality of life for many. However, this integration will be accompanied by significant challenges and risks, including job displacement, ethical concerns, security threats, and geopolitical tensions. The balance of probabilities suggests a future where AI brings both remarkable benefits and substantial uncertainties. Ongoing vigilance, ethical governance, and proactive adaptation will be essential to harness AI's potential while mitigating its risks.

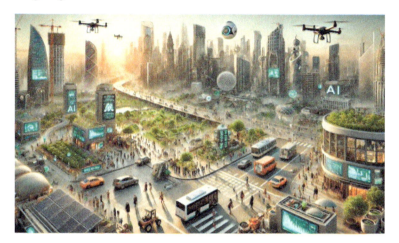

Figure 2 - An image of the world in 2045, reflecting a balance of advancements and challenges in AI. The cityscape shows both modern and dilapidated areas, illustrating economic disparities and the mixed impact of technological progress. Created using DALL-E.

This scenario paints a much scarier picture of the very near future!

Chapter 25: Preparing for this Future

I asked ChatGPT to advise how a father of 3 young children could best prepare them for success in the world of 2045 – this was its recommendation (they seem like very reasonable suggestions to me):

In the scenario of 2045 where AI has significantly impacted society, balancing advancements and challenges, a father of three young children can take several proactive steps to prepare them for success. Here's some advice:

1. Emphasize Lifelong Learning and Adaptability

Encourage Curiosity and Learning: Instil a love of learning in your children. Encourage them to ask questions, explore new topics, and seek knowledge beyond their formal education.

Adaptability Skills: Teach your children to be adaptable and resilient in the face of change. This will help them navigate the rapid technological advancements and shifting job landscapes.

2. Focus on STEM and Beyond

STEM Education: Ensure your children have a strong foundation in science, technology, engineering, and mathematics (STEM). These fields will continue to be critical in a tech-driven world.

Interdisciplinary Skills: Encourage learning in arts, humanities, and social sciences as well. Creativity, critical thinking, and emotional intelligence will be highly valuable.

3. Develop Technological Literacy

Digital Skills: Teach your children to be proficient with current technologies and familiar with emerging ones. Understanding how to use and interact with AI, coding, and digital tools will be essential.

Cybersecurity Awareness: Educate your children about the importance of cybersecurity and how to protect their personal information online.

4. Cultivate Soft Skills and Emotional Intelligence

Communication Skills: Ensure your children are effective communicators, both in writing and speaking. The ability to convey ideas clearly and collaborate with others will be crucial.

Empathy and Teamwork: Encourage empathy, teamwork, and interpersonal skills. These human traits will complement technological skills and be highly sought after in the workforce.

5. Promote Ethical Thinking and Responsibility

Ethical Understanding: Teach your children about the ethical implications of AI and technology. Encourage them to think critically about how technology affects society and their role in shaping its future.

Social Responsibility: Instill a sense of social responsibility. Encourage them to use their skills and knowledge to contribute positively to society and address global challenges like climate change and inequality.

6. Encourage Creativity and Innovation

Creative Pursuits: Support your children in pursuing creative hobbies and interests. Creativity will be a key differentiator in a world where AI handles routine tasks.

Innovative Thinking: Encourage them to think outside the box and come up with innovative solutions to problems. Foster an entrepreneurial mindset.

7. Support Mental and Physical Well-being

Physical Health: Ensure your children stay active and healthy. Regular exercise, proper nutrition, and sufficient sleep are vital for overall well-being.

Mental Health: Promote mental health awareness and provide support. Teach stress management techniques and ensure they have a balanced life.

8. Financial Literacy

Money Management: Educate your children about managing finances, saving, and investing. Financial literacy will help them navigate the economic landscape of the future.

Entrepreneurial Skills: Encourage entrepreneurial thinking and skills. Understanding how to start and manage a business can provide financial independence and opportunities.

9. Engage with Global Perspectives

Cultural Awareness: Expose your children to different cultures and global perspectives. Understanding diverse viewpoints will be valuable in an interconnected world.

Language Skills: Encourage learning multiple languages. Being multilingual can open up global opportunities and enhance cognitive abilities.

10. Stay Informed and Involved

Parental Involvement: Stay informed about technological trends and advancements. Involve yourself in your children's education and extracurricular activities.

Advocacy: Advocate for educational reforms and policies that support technological literacy, ethical AI use, and holistic development in schools.

By fostering a well-rounded education, promoting adaptability, and encouraging ethical and creative thinking, you can help prepare your children to thrive in the complex and evolving world of 2045.

Work to do!

SECTION 6 – GLOSSARY, AI INFLUENCERS & LEADING AI TOOLS

Glossary of Terms for All Things AI

A

- AGI (Artificial General Intelligence): A level of artificial intelligence that can understand, learn, and apply knowledge across a wide range of tasks, mirroring the cognitive abilities of a human being

- API (Application Programming Interface): a set of rules, protocols, and tools that allow different software applications to communicate with each other. APIs enable developers to access specific features or data from a service, system, or application without needing to understand its underlying code or infrastructure. APIs serve as an intermediary, facilitating interactions and data exchanges between different software components, making it easier to build and integrate applications efficiently.

- Algorithm: A step-by-step procedure or formula for solving a problem, typically used in data processing and calculation.

- Artificial Intelligence (AI): The simulation of human intelligence in machines that are programmed to think and learn.

- Artificial Neural Network (ANN): A computational model inspired by the way biological neural networks in the human brain process information.

- Autonomous Systems: Machines or software that can perform tasks without human intervention.

B

- Bias: Systematic errors in data or algorithms that lead to unfair outcomes, often reflecting societal prejudices.

- Big Data: Large and complex data sets that traditional data processing applications cannot handle efficiently.

C

- Chatbot: An AI-powered programme designed to simulate conversation with human users, especially over the internet.

- Computer Vision: A field of AI that enables machines to interpret and make decisions based on visual data from the world.

- Cloud computing: The delivery of computing services, including storage, processing, and software, over the internet, enabling on-demand access to shared resources and applications without the need for local storage infrastructure.

- Convolutional Neural Network (CNN): A type of deep learning model specifically designed to process and analyse and learn from structured grid data, such as images.

D

- Data Mining: The process of discovering patterns and knowledge from large amounts of data.

- Deep Learning: A subset of machine learning involving neural networks with many layers (deep neural networks) that can learn from large amounts of data.

E

- Expert System: A computer system that emulates the decision-making ability of a human expert, often using a set of rules.

- Explainable AI (XAI): Artificial intelligence systems and models that provide clear, understandable, and interpretable explanations of their processes, decisions, and outputs, enabling humans to comprehend, trust, and effectively manage AI systems.

F

- Facial Recognition: A technology capable of identifying or verifying a person from a digital image or a video frame from a video source.

G

- Generative Adversarial Network (GAN): A class of machine learning frameworks where two neural networks, a generator and a discriminator, contest with each other in a game.

- General AI: A type of AI that can understand, learn, and apply knowledge in a general, human-like way across a wide range of tasks.

H

- Hallucination: In the context of AI, particularly with language models, hallucination refers to the generation of output or information that is incorrect, nonsensical, or fabricated. This occurs when the AI produces responses that are not based on its training data or real-world facts, often misleading users with plausible but false information.

- Heuristic: A technique designed to solve a problem faster when classic methods are too slow, by trading optimality, completeness, accuracy, or precision for speed.

I

- Intelligent Agent: An autonomous entity which observes and acts upon an environment and directs its activity towards achieving goals.

- Internet of Things (IoT): The interconnection via the internet of computing devices embedded in everyday objects, enabling them to send and receive data.

J

- Joint Attention: In AI, the shared focus of two or more agents on an object, important for collaborative tasks and social interaction.

K

- Knowledge Base: A technology used to store complex structured and unstructured information used by a computer system.

L

- Learning Algorithm: An algorithm that allows a machine to learn from data and improve its performance over time.

M

- Machine Learning (ML): A type of AI that allows software applications to become more accurate at predicting outcomes without being explicitly programmed.

- Model: In AI, a model is a mathematical representation of a real-world process, trained on data to make predictions or decisions.

N

- Natural Language Processing (NLP): A field of AI that focuses on the interaction between computers and humans through natural language.

- Neural Network: A series of algorithms that attempt to recognise underlying relationships in a set of data through a process that mimics the way the human brain operates.

- Neuromorphic Computing: An approach to designing computer systems inspired by the structure and function of the human brain, utilising specialised hardware and algorithms to mimic neural networks and synapses for more efficient processing, learning, and pattern recognition.

O

- Optimisation: The process of making a system or decision as effective or functional as possible.

P

- Predictive Analytics: The use of data, statistical algorithms, and machine learning techniques to identify the likelihood of future outcomes based on historical data.

- Privacy: In AI, the consideration of safeguarding personal data from unauthorised access and ensuring the ethical use of data.

Q

- Quantum Computing: An area of computing focused on developing computer technology based on the principles of quantum theory, which explains the nature and behavior of energy and matter on the quantum (atomic and subatomic) level.

R

- Reinforcement Learning (RL): A type of machine learning where an agent learns to make decisions by taking actions in an environment to maximise cumulative reward.

- Robotics: The field of AI focused on the design, construction, operation, and use of robots.

S

- Supervised Learning: A type of machine learning where the model is trained on labeled data, meaning the input comes with the correct output.

- Swarm Intelligence: A branch of AI based on the collective behavior of decentralised, self-organised systems, typically natural, such as ant colonies or bird flocking.

T

- Transformer Architecture: A type of deep learning model introduced in the paper "Attention Is All You Need" by Vaswani et al. in 2017. It has revolutionised the field of natural language processing (NLP) and other domains by significantly improving the ability to process and generate human language. It is the foundation of GPTs.

- Turing Test: A test of a machine's ability to exhibit intelligent behavior indistinguishable from that of a human.

U

- Universal Basic Income: A social welfare policy in which all citizens of a country receive a regular, unconditional sum of money from the government regardless of employment status, income level, or other factors. The goal of UBI is to provide financial security, reduce poverty, and address income inequality by ensuring that everyone has a basic level of income to cover essential needs, such as food, housing, and healthcare.

- Unsupervised Learning: A type of machine learning where the model is trained on unlabeled data and must find patterns and relationships in the data.

V

- Virtual Assistant: An AI system that can perform tasks or services for an individual based on commands or questions.

W

- Weak AI: Also known as narrow AI, it is AI that is designed and trained for a specific task, such as voice assistants like Siri or Alexa.

X

- Explainable AI (XAI): AI systems that can provide understandable and interpretable explanations for their decisions and actions.

Z

- Zero-Shot Learning: A type of machine learning where the model can correctly make predictions for new, unseen classes without having been specifically trained on them.

Most Influential People in the AI Industry

(Source: ChatGPT July 2024)

1. Demis Hassabis

- **Current Employment**: CEO and Co-Founder of DeepMind, a subsidiary of Alphabet Inc.

- **Areas of Focus**: Demis Hassabis is focused on developing general AI technologies and applying AI to solve complex scientific challenges. His work at DeepMind includes notable projects such as AlphaGo, AlphaFold (protein folding), and AI applications in healthcare.

2. Andrew Ng

- **Current Employment**: Co-Founder of Coursera and CEO of Landing AI

- **Areas of Focus**: Andrew Ng focuses on democratising access to AI education through Coursera and helping companies implement AI technologies through Landing AI. His work emphasises practical AI applications in industry and education.

3. Fei-Fei Li

- **Current Employment**: Professor at Stanford University and Co-Director of the Stanford Human-Centered AI Institute

- **Areas of Focus**: Fei-Fei Li's research centers on computer vision, cognitive neuroscience, and human-centered AI. She advocates for ethical AI development and improving AI's understanding of human behavior and needs.

Our AI Journey

4. Yann LeCun

- **Current Employment**: Chief AI Scientist at Facebook (Meta) and Professor at New York University

- **Areas of Focus**: Yann LeCun is known for his pioneering work in deep learning and convolutional neural networks. At Facebook, he focuses on advancing AI research and developing AI systems for social media and other applications.

5. Geoffrey Hinton

- **Current Employment**: Emeritus Professor at the University of Toronto and Engineering Fellow at Google

- **Areas of Focus**: Geoffrey Hinton, often referred to as the "Godfather of Deep Learning," continues to work on neural networks and deep learning at Google. His research aims to improve AI's learning algorithms and understanding of neural computation.

6. Elon Musk

- **Current Employment**: CEO of Tesla, SpaceX, and Neuralink; Co-Founder of OpenAI

- **Areas of Focus**: Elon Musk's involvement in AI spans autonomous vehicles at Tesla, brain-computer interfaces at Neuralink, and AI research at OpenAI. He is an advocate for AI safety and ethical considerations in AI development.

7. Sam Altman

- **Current Employment**: CEO of OpenAI

- **Areas of Focus**: Sam Altman leads OpenAI's efforts to ensure that artificial general intelligence (AGI) benefits all of humanity.

He focuses on developing safe and robust AI technologies and promoting their ethical use.

8. Daphne Koller

- **Current Employment**: CEO and Founder of insitro

- **Areas of Focus**: Daphne Koller's work at insitro involves using machine learning and AI to revolutionise drug discovery and development. Her focus is on integrating data science with biology to create new therapeutic insights.

9. Kai-Fu Lee

- **Current Employment**: CEO of Sinovation Ventures and President of Sinovation Ventures Artificial Intelligence Institute

- **Areas of Focus**: Kai-Fu Lee is a prominent AI investor and advocate, focusing on AI innovation and entrepreneurship in China. His work includes fostering AI startups and promoting AI's role in transforming industries.

10. Andrew Moore

- **Current Employment**: Head of Google Cloud AI and former Dean of Carnegie Mellon University's School of Computer Science

- **Areas of Focus**: Andrew Moore's work at Google Cloud AI involves developing AI and machine learning solutions for enterprise applications. His focus includes cloud-based AI services and integrating AI into business processes.

11. Ruslan Salakhutdinov

- **Current Employment**: Director of AI Research at Apple and Professor at Carnegie Mellon University

- **Areas of Focus**: Ruslan Salakhutdinov's research includes deep learning, reinforcement learning, and probabilistic graphical models. At Apple, he leads efforts to integrate advanced AI technologies into consumer products.

12. Ilya Sutskever

- **Current Employment**: Co-Founder and Chief Scientist at OpenAI

- **Areas of Focus**: Ilya Sutskever focuses on developing AGI and advancing the understanding of deep learning. His work includes creating state-of-the-art AI models and ensuring their safe deployment.

13. Pieter Abbeel

- **Current Employment**: Professor at UC Berkeley and Co-Founder of Covariant

- **Areas of Focus**: Pieter Abbeel's research interests include robotics, reinforcement learning, and unsupervised learning. At Covariant, he focuses on applying AI to robotics and automation in industrial settings.

14. Ginni Rometty

- **Current Employment**: Former CEO of IBM, Executive Chairman until her retirement in 2020

- **Areas of Focus**: Under Ginni Rometty's leadership, IBM focused on AI through its Watson platform, which aimed to integrate AI across industries including healthcare, finance, and customer service.

15. Timnit Gebru

- **Current Employment**: Co-Founder of the Distributed AI Research Institute (DAIR)

- **Areas of Focus**: Timnit Gebru's work focuses on ethical AI, algorithmic bias, and the social impacts of AI. At DAIR, she advocates for inclusive and equitable AI research practices.

16. Zoubin Ghahramani

- **Current Employment**: Chief Scientist at Uber

- **Areas of Focus**: Zoubin Ghahramani focuses on machine learning, probabilistic modeling, and AI applications in transportation. His work at Uber involves developing AI systems to optimise ride-sharing, autonomous vehicles, and logistics.

17. Anima Anandkumar

- **Current Employment**: Director of Machine Learning Research at NVIDIA and Professor at Caltech

- **Areas of Focus**: Anima Anandkumar's research spans tensor algebra, deep learning, and AI for scientific applications. She works on developing scalable AI algorithms and applying them to problems in physics, climate science, and healthcare.

18. Jeff Dean

- **Current Employment**: Senior Fellow at Google and Head of Google AI

- **Areas of Focus**: Jeff Dean leads Google's AI division, focusing on advancing deep learning, natural language processing, and AI hardware. His work includes developing AI models like BERT and enhancing AI capabilities across Google's products.

19. Celeste Kidd

- **Current Employment**: Associate Professor of Psychology at UC Berkeley

- **Areas of Focus**: Celeste Kidd's research focuses on cognitive science and how humans, especially children, learn. She investigates the implications of AI on human learning and cognition, emphasising ethical AI in educational tools.

20. Raquel Urtasun

- **Current Employment**: CEO and Founder of Waabi and Professor at the University of Toronto

- **Areas of Focus**: Raquel Urtasun specialises in autonomous driving and computer vision. Her work at Waabi involves developing AI technologies for safer and more efficient self-driving cars.

21. Kate Crawford

- **Current Employment**: Senior Principal Researcher at Microsoft Research and Visiting Professor at MIT

- **Areas of Focus**: Kate Crawford's research focuses on the social and political impacts of AI. She explores issues of data privacy, surveillance, and the ethical implications of AI in society.

22. Hanna Wallach

- **Current Employment**: Principal Researcher at Microsoft Research

- **Areas of Focus**: Hanna Wallach's work centers on machine learning, computational social science, and AI ethics. She investigates how AI systems can be designed to support fairness, accountability, and transparency.

23. Joelle Pineau

- **Current Employment**: Co-Managing Director at Facebook AI Research (FAIR) and Professor at McGill University

- **Areas of Focus**: Joelle Pineau focuses on reinforcement learning, robotics, and healthcare applications of AI. Her research aims to create AI systems that can learn and adapt to complex environments.

24. Chris Urmson

- **Current Employment**: CEO and Co-Founder of Aurora Innovation

- **Areas of Focus**: Chris Urmson is a leading figure in autonomous vehicles. At Aurora, he works on developing self-driving technology to improve safety and efficiency in transportation.

25. Tim Hwang

- **Current Employment**: CEO of FiscalNote

- **Areas of Focus**: Tim Hwang's work involves leveraging AI for legal and political analytics. He focuses on using AI to analyse legislation, regulatory data, and provide insights for policy-making.

26. Lila Ibrahim

- **Current Employment**: COO of DeepMind

- **Areas of Focus**: Lila Ibrahim oversees operations at DeepMind, focusing on organisational strategy, partnerships, and ensuring that AI research is conducted responsibly and ethically.

27. Margaret Mitchell

- **Current Employment**: Chief Ethics Scientist at Hugging Face

- **Areas of Focus**: Margaret Mitchell works on AI ethics, focusing on fairness, accountability, and transparency in AI systems. She aims to create AI technologies that are equitable and just.

28. Dario Amodei

- **Current Employment**: CEO and Co-Founder of Anthropic

- **Areas of Focus**: Dario Amodei's work at Anthropic focuses on creating safe and aligned AI systems. He aims to develop AI technologies that are beneficial and controllable, addressing potential risks associated with AI.

29. Ian Goodfellow

- **Current Employment**: Director of Machine Learning at Apple

- **Areas of Focus**: Ian Goodfellow is known for inventing Generative Adversarial Networks (GANs). His work at Apple involves advancing machine learning algorithms and applying them to enhance Apple's products.

30. Daniela Rus

- **Current Employment**: Director of the Computer Science and Artificial Intelligence Laboratory (CSAIL) at MIT

- **Areas of Focus**: Daniela Rus focuses on robotics, autonomous systems, and AI in manufacturing. Her research aims to create intelligent machines that can operate alongside humans safely and efficiently.

Top 100 Most Significant AI Tools

This list is compiled based on current use levels in 2024 using Chat GPT and includes a variety of tools that span across multiple domains within AI, such as machine learning frameworks, data analysis platforms, natural language processing tools, computer vision libraries, and more. (Generative AI tools are explored in Chapter 2.)

These tools represent a wide array of AI applications and are critical in various sectors, from data science and machine learning to natural language processing, computer vision, and robotics. They are selected based on their widespread use and significance in 2024. Here's the list:

Machine Learning Frameworks

1. **TensorFlow**: Widely used machine learning framework developed by Google.

2. **PyTorch**: Popular deep learning library developed by Facebook.

3. **Scikit-Learn**: Python library for machine learning and data analysis.

4. **Keras**: High-level neural networks API, running on TensorFlow.

5. **XGBoost**: Optimised distributed gradient boosting library.

6. **LightGBM**: Gradient boosting framework that uses tree-based learning algorithms.

7. **H2O.ai**: Open-source platform for AI, machine learning, and predictive analytics.

8. **CatBoost**: High-performance gradient boosting library.

9. **Apache MXNet**: Scalable deep learning framework.

10. **Caffe**: Deep learning framework focused on speed and modularity.

Natural Language Processing (NLP)

11. **NLTK (Natural Language Toolkit)**: Suite of libraries and programmes for symbolic and statistical NLP.

12. **SpaCy**: Open-source library for advanced NLP in Python.

13. **BERT (Bidirectional Encoder Representations from Transformers)**: Pre-trained NLP model by Google.

14. **OpenAI GPT-3**: State-of-the-art language model by OpenAI.

15. **Transformers by Hugging Face**: Library providing thousands of pre-trained models for NLP.

16. **AllenNLP**: Open-source NLP research library built on PyTorch.

17. **Stanford NLP**: Suite of NLP tools developed by the Stanford NLP Group.

18. **TextBlob**: Simple library for processing textual data in Python.

19. **Gensim**: Library for topic modeling and document similarity analysis.

20. **Flair**: Simple NLP library for state-of-the-art natural language processing.

Computer Vision

21. **OpenCV**: Library of programming functions for real-time computer vision.

22. **YOLO (You Only Look Once)**: Real-time object detection system.

23. **Detectron2**: Facebook AI Research library for object detection and segmentation.

24. **TensorFlow Object Detection API**: Framework for building and training object detection models.

25. **Dlib**: Toolkit for machine learning and data analysis, including face detection.

26. **KerasCV**: Keras-based tools for computer vision tasks.

27. **Mediapipe**: Framework for building multimodal, applied ML pipelines.

28. **VGGFace**: Deep learning library for face recognition tasks.

29. **DeepFaceLab**: Open-source deepfake system.

30. **Face++**: Facial recognition and analysis service.

Reinforcement Learning

31. **OpenAI Gym**: Toolkit for developing and comparing reinforcement learning algorithms.

32. **Stable Baselines3**: Set of improved implementations of reinforcement learning algorithms.

33. **RLlib**: Scalable reinforcement learning library built on Ray.

34. **DeepMind Lab**: 3D learning environment for agent-based AI research.

35. **Unity ML-Agents**: Toolkit for training intelligent agents using Unity.

36. **TensorForce**: Reinforcement learning library built on TensorFlow.

37. **RoboSchool**: Environments for reinforcement learning in robotics.

38. **Acme**: Research framework for reinforcement learning.

39. **Maze**: Scalable reinforcement learning library for large-scale applications.

40. **Coach**: Reinforcement learning research framework.

Automated Machine Learning (AutoML)

41. **AutoML by Google Cloud**: Suite of machine learning products that enable developers with limited expertise to train high-quality models.

42. **Auto-sklearn**: Open-source library for AutoML.

43. **H2O AutoML**: Tool for automating the machine learning workflow.

44. **TPOT**: Automated machine learning library for Python.

45. **DataRobot**: AI-driven enterprise AutoML platform.

46. **MLJar**: AutoML for advanced machine learning and interpretability.

47. **TransmogrifAI**: AutoML library for structured data.

48. **Featuretools**: Open-source library for automated feature engineering.

49. **BigML**: Machine learning platform for AutoML.

50. **Microsoft Azure AutoML**: Automated machine learning service by Microsoft Azure.

Data Visualisation

51. **Tableau**: Powerful data visualisation tool used for data analysis and business intelligence.

52. **Power BI**: Business analytics service by Microsoft.

53. **Plotly**: Open-source graphing library that makes interactive, publication-quality graphs online.

54. **D3.js**: JavaScript library for producing dynamic, interactive data visualisations in web browsers.

55. **Matplotlib**: Comprehensive library for creating static, animated, and interactive visualisations in Python.

56. **Seaborn**: Python data visualisation library based on Matplotlib.

57. **ggplot2**: Data visualisation package for the R programming language.

58. **QlikView**: Business intelligence and data visualisation tool.

59. **Looker**: Data exploration and discovery business intelligence platform.

60. **Sisense**: Business intelligence software for data visualisation and analysis.

Data Integration and ETL

61. **Apache Kafka**: Distributed event streaming platform capable of handling real-time data feeds.

62. **Apache Spark**: Unified analytics engine for large-scale data processing.

63. **Talend**: Data integration tool for ETL processes.

64. **Alteryx**: Data blending and advanced data analytics tool.

65. **Informatica**: Data integration software.

66. **Pentaho**: Business intelligence and data integration software.

67. **Fivetran**: Data integration tool for ETL.

68. **Stitch**: Simple, extensible ETL service for data integration.

69. **Dataiku**: Data science and machine learning platform.

70. **Knime**: Open-source data analytics, reporting, and integration platform.

AI for Business and Productivity

71. **Salesforce Einstein**: AI platform that powers predictions and recommendations for customer relationship management.

72. **IBM Watson**: Suite of AI tools for business, including NLP, machine learning, and computer vision.

73. **Azure Machine Learning**: Cloud-based environment for training, deploying, and managing machine learning models.

74. **Google Cloud AI**: Suite of machine learning products and tools provided by Google Cloud.

75. **AWS SageMaker**: Fully managed service that provides every developer and data scientist with the ability to build, train, and deploy machine learning models.

76. **UiPath**: Robotic process automation tool that uses AI to automate repetitive tasks.

77. **Automation Anywhere**: AI-powered robotic process automation tool.

78. **CognitiveScale**: AI software for industry-specific solutions.

79. **Blue Prism**: Robotic process automation software.

80. **H2O Driverless AI**: Enterprise AI platform for building and deploying machine learning models.

AI in Robotics

81. **ROS (Robot Operating System)**: Flexible framework for writing robot software.

82. **V-REP (CoppeliaSim)**: Versatile and scalable robot simulation software.

83. **MoveIt**: Software for mobile manipulation in robotics.

84. **Gazebo**: Open-source 3D robotics simulator.

85. **RoboDK**: Simulation and offline programming software for industrial robots.

86. **Webots**: Open-source robot simulator.

87. **Choreonoid**: Integrated robotics development environment.

88. **Marvin AI**: Platform for building AI-powered robots.

89. **Autoware**: Open-source software for autonomous driving.

90. **Aido**: AI and robotics platform for building intelligent robots.

Miscellaneous AI Tools

91. **Claude**: Conversational AI model by Anthropic.

92. **GPT-3 Playground**: Interface to interact with OpenAI's GPT-3 for generating text.

93. **DeepArt.io**: AI-powered tool for transforming photos into artworks using deep neural networks.

94. **Grammarly**: AI-powered writing assistant that helps correct grammar, punctuation, and style.

95. **Hugging Face's Transformers**: Library providing thousands of pre-trained models for NLP.

96. **IBM Project Debater**: AI system that can engage in debate with humans on complex topics.

97. **SAS Viya**: Cloud-enabled, in-memory analytics engine for AI and machine learning.

98. **Wit.ai**: Natural language interface for applications capable of turning speech and text into actionable data.

99. **Dialogflow**: Google's platform for building conversational interfaces using NLP.

100.**NVIDIA DeepStream**: AI-powered video analytics toolkit.

Conversational AI Agents

Conversational AI agents are intelligent systems designed to interact with humans through natural language, using technologies such as natural language processing (NLP), machine learning, and speech recognition to understand, respond to, and engage in human-like conversations across various platforms.

- **Google Assistant**
    - ○ **Developed by**: Google
    - ○ **Capabilities**: Voice interaction, search, scheduling, device control, contextual conversation, smart home integration.

- **Amazon Alexa**
    - ○ **Developed by**: Amazon
    - ○ **Capabilities**: Voice interaction, music playback, making to-do lists, setting alarms, streaming podcasts, smart home device control.

- **Apple Siri**
    - ○ **Developed by**: Apple
    - ○ **Capabilities**: Voice commands, text-based commands, information retrieval, device control, messaging, smart home integration.

- **Microsoft Cortana**
    - ○ **Developed by**: Microsoft
    - ○ **Capabilities**: Voice commands, search, productivity tasks, reminders, smart home integration.

Our AI Journey

- **Samsung Bixby**

    - **Developed by**: Samsung

    - **Capabilities**: Voice interaction, device control, contextual understanding, smart home integration.

Customer Service and Support AI Agents

Customer Service and Support Agents are automated systems dedicated to assisting customers by addressing their inquiries, resolving issues, and providing information about products or services to ensure customer satisfaction and support.

- **IBM Watson Assistant**

    - **Developed by**: IBM

    - **Capabilities**: Natural language processing, conversational AI, customer service automation, chatbot capabilities.

- **Zendesk Answer Bot**

    - **Developed by**: Zendesk

    - **Capabilities**: Customer service automation, knowledge base integration, natural language processing.

- **Intercom Custom Bots**

    - **Developed by**: Intercom

    - **Capabilities**: Customer engagement, lead qualification, conversational AI.

- **Ada**

    - **Developed by**: Ada

    - **Capabilities**: Automated customer support, natural language understanding, multi-channel integration.

- **Bold360**

    - **Developed by**: LogMeIn

    - **Capabilities**: AI chatbots, customer engagement, natural language processing.

Virtual Personal Assistants

Virtual Personal Assistants are AI-powered software applications designed to help users with a variety of tasks, such as managing schedules, providing information, sending messages, and performing other personal or professional activities, by understanding and responding to natural language commands.

- **x.ai**

    - **Developed by**: x.ai

    - **Capabilities**: Scheduling meetings, calendar management, email integration.

- **Clara**

    - **Developed by**: Clara Labs

    - **Capabilities**: Meeting scheduling, email handling, natural language processing.

- **Zoom.ai**
  - **Developed by**: Zoom.ai
  - **Capabilities**: Meeting scheduling, task automation, knowledge retrieval.

- **Julie Desk**
  - **Developed by**: Julie Desk
  - **Capabilities**: Email management, meeting scheduling, calendar coordination.

AI Agents for Business and Productivity

AI Agents for Business and Productivity are artificial intelligence-driven tools designed to enhance efficiency and performance in business operations by automating tasks, analysing data, managing workflows, and providing insights to support decision-making and increase overall productivity.

- **Salesforce Einstein**
  - **Developed by**: Salesforce
  - **Capabilities**: AI for CRM, predictive analytics, customer insights, natural language processing.

- **Zoho Zia**
  - **Developed by**: Zoho
  - **Capabilities**: AI-powered CRM, sales prediction, customer insights, natural language processing.

- **HubSpot AI**

  - **Developed by**: HubSpot

  - **Capabilities**: Marketing automation, sales insights, customer service, conversational AI.

Specialised AI Agents

Specialised AI Agents are artificial intelligence systems designed to perform specific tasks or functions within a particular domain or industry, leveraging advanced algorithms and domain-specific knowledge to deliver optimised and highly effective solutions for targeted applications.

- **Replika**

  - **Developed by**: Luka, Inc.

  - **Capabilities**: AI companionship, emotional support, conversational AI.

- **Mitsuku**

  - **Developed by**: Steve Worswick, Pandorabots

  - **Capabilities**: General conversation, Turing Test winner, natural language understanding.

- **Woebot**

  - **Developed by**: Woebot Labs

  - **Capabilities**: Mental health support, cognitive behavioural therapy, conversational AI.

- **ELIZA**

  - **Developed by**: Joseph Weizenbaum

- Capabilities: Early natural language processing, simulates a Rogerian psychotherapist.

AI Agents for Autonomous Systems

AI Agents for Autonomous Systems are intelligent systems designed to operate independently without human intervention, using machine learning and other AI technologies to make decisions, navigate, and perform tasks in dynamic environments, such as self-driving cars, drones, and robotic systems.

- **Tesla Autopilot**
    - **Developed by**: Tesla
    - **Capabilities**: Autonomous driving, driver assistance, real-time navigation, computer vision.

- **Waymo Driver**
    - **Developed by**: Waymo (Alphabet Inc.)
    - **Capabilities**: Fully autonomous driving, real-time navigation, computer vision, AI-based decision making.

- **Nuro**
    - **Developed by**: Nuro
    - **Capabilities**: Autonomous delivery vehicles, real-time navigation, computer vision.

- **Cruise**
    - **Developed by**: Cruise (General Motors)

- Capabilities: Fully autonomous driving, real-time navigation, computer vision.

AI Agents in Healthcare

AI Agents in Healthcare are advanced AI-driven systems designed to assist in medical tasks, such as diagnosing diseases, recommending treatments, managing patient records, and providing personalised care, by analysing complex medical data and enhancing decision-making processes for healthcare professionals.

- **Babylon Health**
    - Developed by: Babylon Health
    - Capabilities: Symptom checking, telehealth, AI diagnostics.

- **Buoy Health**
    - Developed by: Buoy Health
    - Capabilities: Symptom checking, personalised health information, AI diagnostics.

- **Ada Health**
    - Developed by: Ada Health
    - Capabilities: Symptom assessment, health guidance, AI diagnostics.

- **Sensely**
    - Developed by: Sensely

- Capabilities: Virtual nurse assistant, patient monitoring, symptom assessment.

- **K Health**

  - **Developed by**: K Health

  - **Capabilities**: Symptom checking, telehealth, personalised health information.

AI Agents for Finance

AI Agents for Finance are intelligent systems that leverage advanced algorithms and machine learning to perform tasks such as fraud detection, algorithmic trading, risk assessment, customer service, and financial forecasting, thereby enhancing efficiency, accuracy, and decision-making in financial services.

- **Kavout**

  - **Developed by**: Kavout

  - **Capabilities**: AI for investment analysis, predictive analytics, stock scoring.

- **AlphaSense**

  - **Developed by**: AlphaSense

  - **Capabilities**: AI for financial research, market intelligence, data analytics.

- **Kensho**

  - **Developed by**: S&P Global

- o **Capabilities**: Financial analytics, predictive modeling, data visualisation.

- **ZestFinance**

  - o **Developed by**: Zest AI

  - o **Capabilities**: AI-driven credit scoring, risk management, financial analytics.

- **Tink**

  - o **Developed by**: Tink

  - o **Capabilities**: Open banking, financial data aggregation, AI-driven financial insights.

Miscellaneous AI Agents

Miscellaneous AI Agents are a diverse group of artificial intelligence systems designed to perform a variety of specialised tasks across different domains that do not fall under conventional categories, including applications in entertainment, education, agriculture, and more, each tailored to meet specific needs and enhance various aspects of daily life and industry.

- **OpenAI Codex**

  - o **Developed by**: OpenAI

  - o **Capabilities**: Code generation, programming assistance, natural language understanding.

- **Copilot**

  - o **Developed by**: GitHub and OpenAI

- $\circ$ **Capabilities**: Code suggestions, programming assistance, natural language processing.

- **AlphaFold**

  - $\circ$ **Developed by**: DeepMind

  - $\circ$ **Capabilities**: Protein folding prediction, bioinformatics, structural biology.

- **DALL-E**

  - $\circ$ **Developed by**: OpenAI

  - $\circ$ **Capabilities**: Image generation from textual descriptions, creative AI, visual art.

- **Jasper (formerly Jarvis)**

  - $\circ$ **Developed by**: Jasper.ai

  - $\circ$ **Capabilities**: AI content generation, copywriting, creative writing.

AI Agents for Personal Use

AI Agents for Personal Use are intelligent systems designed to assist individuals with everyday tasks, such as managing schedules, organising personal information, providing recommendations, controlling smart home devices, and facilitating communication, by understanding and responding to natural language commands and preferences.

- **Replika**

  - $\circ$ **Developed by**: Luka, Inc.

- Capabilities: AI companionship, conversational AI, emotional support.

- **Mycroft**

  - **Developed by**: Mycroft AI

  - **Capabilities**: Open-source voice assistant, smart home integration, conversational AI.

- **Jibo**

  - **Developed by**: Jibo, Inc.

  - **Capabilities**: Social robot, personal assistant, smart home integration.

- **Misa**

  - **Developed by**: Misa Robotics

  - **Capabilities**: Social robot, personal assistant, educational companion.

AI Agents for Entertainment

AI Agents for Entertainment are intelligent systems designed to enhance user experiences in media and leisure activities by creating, curating, and recommending content, interacting with users through games and virtual environments, and personalising entertainment options based on user preferences and behaviour.

- **Suki AI**

  - **Developed by**: Suki AI

  - **Capabilities**: AI assistant for healthcare providers, voice-enabled medical documentation.

- **Cortexica**
  - **Developed by**: Cortexica Vision Systems
  - **Capabilities**: Visual search, image recognition, fashion and retail applications.

- **Synthesia**
  - **Developed by**: Synthesia
  - **Capabilities**: AI video generation, virtual presenters, video content creation.

- **Aiva**
  - **Developed by**: Aiva Technologies
  - **Capabilities**: AI music composition, virtual composer, creative AI.

- **Lobe**
  - **Developed by**: Microsoft
  - **Capabilities**: Simple machine learning model creation, visual interface, AI training.

- **Replica Studios**
  - **Developed by**: Replica Studios
  - **Capabilities**: AI voice acting, synthetic voices, entertainment and gaming.

These AI agents represent a diverse range of applications, from personal assistants and customer service bots to specialised tools in healthcare, finance, and creative industries. They are significant in their respective fields due to their advanced capabilities and widespread adoption.

REFERENCES

Reference Number	Source	Pages Used/Applicable Sections
1	Alan Turing, "Computing Machinery and Intelligence," *Mind* 59, no. 236 (1950): 433-460.	History of AI – Alan Turing and the Turing Test
2	John McCarthy et al., "A Proposal for the Dartmouth Summer Research Project on Artificial Intelligence" (1956).	The Dartmouth Conference and AI establishment
3	Herbert A. Simon and Allen Newell, *The Logic Theorist: Human Problem Solving* (1963).	Early AI Development – Logic Theorist
4	Frank Rosenblatt, "The Perceptron: A Perceiving and Recognizing Automaton," *Cornell Aeronautical Laboratory Report* (1957).	Perceptron and Neural Networks
5	Joseph Welzenbaum, *ELIZA – A Computer Program for the Study of Natural Language Communication between Man and Machine* (1966).	Natural Language Processing, ELIZA
6	Geoffrey Hinton, David Rumelhart, and Ronald Williams, "Learning Representations by Back-propagating Errors," *Nature* 323 (1986): 533-536.	Backpropagation and Neural Networks

Reference Number	Source	Pages Used/Applicable Sections
7	Fei-Fei Li et al., "ImageNet: A Large-Scale Hierarchical Image Database," *Computer Vision and Pattern Recognition* (2009).	ImageNet and AlexNet, Breakthrough in Computer Vision
8	Alex Krizhevsky, Ilya Sutskever, and Geoffrey Hinton, "ImageNet Classification with Deep Convolutional Neural Networks," *Advances in Neural Information Processing Systems* (2012).	CNN and Deep Learning – ImageNet Results
9	Demis Hassabis, "AlphaGo," *Nature* (2016).	AlphaGo – Reinforcement Learning and Game AI
10	OpenAI, "GPT-3: Language Models are Few-Shot Learners," *arXiv preprint* (2020).	Natural Language Processing and GPT-3
11	Elon Musk, "Tesla Full Self-Driving and the Future of Autonomous Vehicles," *Tesla Investor Day Speech* (2022).	Autonomous Vehicles and AI
12	Nick Bostrom, *Superintelligence: Paths, Dangers, Strategies* (Oxford University Press, 2014).	AGI, Existential Risks of AI
13	Stuart Russell and Peter Norvig, *Artificial Intelligence: A Modern Approach* (Pearson, 2021).	General AI Theories, Concepts, and History

Reference Number	Source	Pages Used/Applicable Sections
14	Gary Marcus and Ernest Davis, *Rebooting AI: Building Artificial Intelligence We Can Trust* (Pantheon, 2019).	Ethical Concerns and Trust in AI
15	DALL-E by OpenAI, official API documentation.	Text-to-Image Tools
16	MidJourney, official tool description.	Text-to-Image Tools
17	Synthesia, official product description.	Text-to-Video Tools
18	Pictory AI, company documentation.	Text-to-Video Tools
19	Elon Musk, Sam Altman, and Demis Hassabis, interviews on AGI and AI governance, *Future of Humanity Institute Podcast* (2021).	AI Governance and AGI Prospects
20	Stuart Russell, "Human Compatible: AI and the Problem of Control" (Viking, 2019).	Safety, Control, and Ethical Concerns
21	Timnit Gebru, "Race and Gender in AI: Ethical Issues and Solutions," *AI Ethics Journal* (2018).	Bias and Fairness in AI
22	Shoshana Zuboff, *The Age of Surveillance Capitalism* (PublicAffairs, 2019).	AI and Privacy Concerns, Surveillance

Reference Number	Source	Pages Used/Applicable Sections
23	Fei-Fei Li, "The Future of AI in Healthcare," *Stanford Medicine* (2021).	AI in Healthcare, Personalized Treatments
24	Erik Brynjolfsson and Andrew McAfee, *The Second Machine Age: Work, Progress, and Prosperity in a Time of Brilliant Technologies* (Norton & Company, 2014).	Economic Impact of AI, Job Displacement
25	Ray Kurzweil, *The Singularity is Near: When Humans Transcend Biology* (Penguin, 2005).	The Future of AI, Technological Singularity
26	Fei-Fei Li and John Etchemendy, "AI and Society: The Role of AI in the 21st Century," *Stanford Human-Centered AI Institute* (2021).	AI's Societal Impact
27	DeepMind, official blog, "AlphaFold: Solving the Protein Folding Problem," (2020).	AI and Scientific Discovery
28	Geoffrey Hinton, "Deep Learning: Past, Present, and Future," *MIT AI Podcast* (2021).	Deep Learning Breakthroughs

Reference Number	Source	Pages Used/Applicable Sections
29	McKinsey Global Institute, "AI in Logistics and Supply Chain," McKinsey Report (2022).	AI in Logistics and Route Optimization
30	PwC, "AI Predictions 2023: Ethics, Adoption, and Regulation," PwC Research Report (2023).	AI Adoption and Regulatory Frameworks
31	Dario Amodei et al., "AI Safety and Alignment: Solving the Control Problem," *OpenAI Blog* (2021).	AI Safety and Alignment Challenges
32	OpenAI Codex, official documentation (2021).	AI in Programming and Development
33	MIT Technology Review, "The Future of AI Governance," (2022).	AI Governance and Policy-Making
34	Karen Hao, "The Race for General AI: Where Are We Now?" *MIT Technology Review* (2021).	AGI Development and Current Status
35	Patrick Winston, *Artificial Intelligence: The MIT View* (MIT Press, 2021).	Overview of AI Concepts and Applications
36	Tesla AI Day presentations (2022).	Autonomous Driving and AI Systems

Reference Number	Source	Pages Used/Applicable Sections
37	Max Tegmark, *Life 3.0: Being Human in the Age of Artificial Intelligence* (Knopf, 2017).	AGI and Future Implications for Human Society
38	Gartner Research, "AI in Business: Trends and Predictions," (2022).	AI in Business and Productivity
39	AI Now Institute, "AI Ethics and Governance in 2023," AI Now Annual Report (2023).	Ethical Concerns and Governance
40	Rob High, "AI at IBM: Watson's Evolution," *IBM AI Research* (2021).	AI in Healthcare, Watson's Development

THE END

Or perhaps the beginning of a journey to ensure that AI is harnessed for the betterment of all humanity and the future of our planet?

Printed in Great Britain
by Amazon